Not Tonight I Have a HEADACHE

Not Tonight I Have a HEADACHE

*Understanding Headache and
Eliminating It From Your Life*

Ravinder Singh, M.D.

New York

Not Tonight I Have a HEADACHE
Understanding Headache and Eliminating It From Your Life

Published in New York, New York, by Morgan James Publishing. Morgan James and The Entrepreneurial Publisher are trademarks of Morgan James, LLC.
www.MorganJamesPublishing.com

The Morgan James Speakers Group can bring authors to your live event. For more information or to book an event visit The Morgan James Speakers Group at
www.TheMorganJamesSpeakersGroup.com.

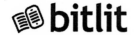

A **free** eBook edition is available
with the purchase of this print book.

CLEARLY PRINT YOUR NAME ABOVE IN UPPER CASE
Instructions to claim your free eBook edition:
1. Download the BitLit app for Android or iOS
2. Write your name in **UPPER CASE** on the line
3. Use the BitLit app to submit a photo
4. Download your eBook to any device

ISBN 978-1-63047-363-1 paperback
ISBN 978-1-63047-364-8 eBook
ISBN 978-1-63047-365-5 hardcover
Library of Congress Control Number:
2014945673

Cover Design by:
Rachel Lopez
www.r2cdesign.com

In an effort to support local communities and raise awareness and funds, Morgan James Publishing donates a percentage of all book sales for the life of each book to Habitat for Humanity Peninsula and Greater Williamsburg.

Get involved today, visit
www.MorganJamesBuilds.com

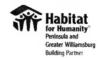

Habitat
for Humanity®
Peninsula and
Greater Williamsburg
Building Partner

Dedicated to all headache sufferers
who desire freedom from pain

Table of Contents

Foreword

I have had the pleasure of knowing Dr. Ravinder Singh since he was a resident-physician in neurology at the Veterans Administration Medical Center in West Los Angeles (VAMC WLA), California, and the University of California, Los Angeles (UCLA) in the mid-1990s. He was just becoming involved with clinical research in neurology, more specifically in the treatment of stroke. He was involved in the initial studies that eventually led to the approval of the first drug to reverse and treat acute ischemic stroke.

Recently, I had the pleasure of working closely with Ravinder when I became the chairman of the department of neurology at Cedars-Sinai Medical Center in Los Angeles. Dr. Singh is a neurologist held in high regard by his colleagues at Cedars-Sinai. In 2012, he was awarded the prestigious Friend of Nursing Award by the Department of Nursing. Recognized for his warmth, knowledge, and collaboration with nurses, Dr. Singh is a valued member of the stroke team.

Dr. Singh has a passion for and knowledge of both Western and Eastern medicine. Western medicine has been slow to embrace the Eastern disciplines, partly because of the notion that they have little basis in the modern world of hypothesis-driven science. The medical profession is dominated by the scientific method, exemplified by the use randomized, controlled trials while ignoring the knowledge acquired through thousands of years of direct observation, introspection, and knowledge of the energetic aspects of disease that are difficult to measure by scientific methodology.

But the West has slowly opened its doors in the last few decades to Eastern medicinal practices such as yoga, acupuncture, homeopathy, chiropractic, and the like. Often we have been led by our patients, perhaps learning about effective treatments that have not been described in traditional Western medical journals. Skeptical scientists are still wary of the concepts of prana or chi. Despite methodological challenges, rigorous scientific studies are slowly making their way into the Eastern field, proving that there is substance to the health claims of these methodologies.

In the same way as the practitioners of the Western sciences look askance at the "non-scientific" approaches of the Eastern disciplines, the proponents of the Eastern disciplines are wary of the scientific methods, touting the superiority of the traditional approaches. Certainly, there are benefits to both and drawbacks of both. Each discipline has strengths and weaknesses. Yet very few individuals are equally comfortable in the practice of both the Western and Eastern disciplines. As we enter the next phase of healthcare, providers will need to study all different types of treatment modalities.

Given the current state of affairs, Dr. Ravinder Singh's *Not Tonight, I Have a Headache: Understanding Headache and Eliminating It from Your Life* is a welcome endeavor. In it, he writes from the perspective of an Eastern practitioner and a physician-scientist trained at one of the best medical institutions of the West. He has set himself the ambitious goal of combining the modern, scientific understanding and treatment of a very common condition, headache, with the various ancient practices of the East.

Dr Singh's interest in headache and the care of the patient with chronic headaches led him to write this book. *Not Tonight, I Have a Headache* is a labor of love. His suggestions and interventions are helpful and safe, and those who suffer chronic headaches will find this book enormously useful.

—**Patrick Lyden, MD.**, Los Angeles, California

Acknowledgments

This book is the product of blessings and grace from the Creator who is the repository of all knowledge.

My heartfelt love and thanks to my wife, Gurmehar Kaur, who was instrumental in helping me create this vision, and for providing me with support in bringing the project to fruition. I would also like to thank my parents, Manmohan Singh and Narinjan Kaur, for their undying love and support.

I especially want to express my appreciation to my patients who provided me the inspiration to help others obtain relief from headache pain.

—**Ravinder Singh, MD.**, Los Angeles, California

Disclaimer

This book is designed to provide information about the subject matter covered. It is sold with the understanding that the authors are not rendering medical advice or other professional services. If medical or other expert assistance is required, the services of a medical professional or other competent health care practitioner should be sought.

It is not the purpose of this manual to be an exhaustive treatise on all available information on the treatment of headaches, but to complement and supplement other available information.

Obtaining freedom from headaches does not depend on a quick fix. Anyone who desires to become headache-free must expect to invest time and effort without any guarantee of success. Reading a book is not going to bring you this freedom. Doing the exercises and creating a different mindset will help you toward achieving that goal.

Every effort has been made to make this book as complete and accurate as possible. However, there may be mistakes of content and typography. This text should be used only as a general guide and not as the ultimate headache resource. As more information becomes available on the different causes and treatments of headache, some information may become obsolete. This book contains current information on headaches as of the date of publication.

The purpose of the book is to educate. The authors and publishers have neither liability nor responsibility to any person or entity with respect to any loss or damage caused or alleged to be caused directly or indirectly by the information contained in this book.

Introduction

"Not tonight, honey, I have a headache." This is probably one of the most common utterances in any household, especially between a husband and wife. But it can take a whole new meaning if you really suffer from headaches. The existence of headache pain is as old as humankind. Only the rare individual can claim to be headache free his entire life. It is surprising that despite the widespread prevalence of headaches, many people do not take them seriously, and every headache sufferer tries remedies, with varying degrees of success, that he or she believes will be effective.

This lack of seriousness has resulted in the increased incidence of headaches for which medical attention is sought. It is one of the three most common conditions for which a neurological consultation is pursued, the other two being dizziness and back pain. In reality, headache can be a serious, debilitating illness. It has the potential to be life altering, and in extreme cases, it affects one's career, school, and social life, and thus one's quality of life overall. Its impact on society is increasing at an alarming rate. Billions of dollars are lost to businesses; thousands of school days are lost per month nationwide. Headaches are the number-one reason for missing work and school, not counting people who go to work despite their headaches, causing them to function at less than their best.

As a neurologist, I have noticed that some patients respond to certain medications while others do not. Many patients referred to me for headache treatment have never seen an improvement in their symptoms through medications. I remember a patient suffering from chronic migraine. Before she was referred to me, she had gone to various doctors who had tried all medications available at that time but with little effect. After talking to her, I realized that the medications were not given to her in the appropriate doses for an appropriate length of time, and the side effects of the medications were perhaps not taken into consideration. I adjusted her medications in a way that maximized pain control while minimizing the side effects.

In much of Western medicine, there is a common knee-jerk reaction: You have a headache? Here, take this pill. Human nature demands instant gratification. People generally are looking for a quick fix to their problems. Catering to this mentality, a myriad of over-the-counter (OTC) remedies can be found in local pharmacies. While these remedies may be effective in controlling the symptoms of headaches, they do not address the cause of the pain.

The question arises then, that if there are so many OTC treatments available, why are people suffering? If the majority of the headaches are benign, why are emergency departments and doctors' offices filled with patients suffering intolerable headaches whose treatments have not eliminated the pain? Why are patients drifting from doctor to doctor, seeking treatments and resigning themselves to suffer needlessly when none is effective? Is this their destiny? With all the resources modern medicine has at its disposal, why is this happening? Is there a flaw in our approach?

Three hundred years ago, Descartes expounded the absolute separation of mind and body. As a result, the practice of medicine took his mechanistic view that science is only concerned with the visible, physical, and material reality, separate from the mind. Scientific research has focused primarily on the physical, on the distinction between mind and body, causing scientists to rely exclusively on observation for their development of mechanistic explanations of physical events. Much of mainstream Western medicine is a product of this reductionist view. As a result, the focus is on the disease and its symptoms, not on overall health and the underlying cause of the disease.

When we explore the medical practices of societies that trace their origins back thousands of years, we see a different picture. Even Socrates stated almost twenty-five hundred years ago that the mind cannot be split from the body. In Plato's dialogues, Socrates states that this is the reason the cure of so many diseases is unknown to the physicians of Hellas; they are ignorant of the whole. This is also the great error of our day in the treatment of the human body: physicians separate the mind from the body.

Chinese traditions of acupuncture, Indian traditions of Ayurvedic medicine and yoga, Islamic traditions, Native American medical practices, and many other healing traditions of different native societies all view the body as a whole. These ancient traditions do not separate the mind from the body but focus mainly on health and cause of disease rather than just the symptoms. Instead of focusing just on the outward manifestations of disease, the practitioners of these ancient arts focus on the elusive underlying cause of the disease and direct their treatments toward that cause.

To illustrate, let me give an example of one such technique. Nambudripad's Allergy Elimination Technique (NAET) addresses the cause of the disease instead of merely attempting to alleviate the symptoms of the allergy sufferer. The NAET technique combines Chinese medicine with other disciplines such as kinesiology, chiropractic treatment, and allergy elimination, among others.

I started incorporating NAET, lifestyle review, and stress management where applicable into my practice with astounding results. Not only were my patients having fewer headaches, but the quality of their life improved as well. Their general health improved. Once I considered the possibility of alternative medicine, I met several alternative practitioners, such as acupuncturists, homeopathic physicians, and chiropractors. It became evident that each had something to offer the headache sufferer.

Eastern medicine is concerned with the whole individual in disease prevention, assessing the factors or combination of factors that led to the symptoms, and addressing those causative factors rather than just camouflaging the symptoms with medications. The focus is on the *cause* rather than the *symptom*. My studies ultimately led me back to my roots, to the teachings of my own religion, Sikhism, where I finally understood the reality behind the mind-body connection. This taught me the core principles to eliminating disease.

I would like the readers to know that I adhere to Sikh spiritual traditions as my faith; hence, when I refer to my spiritual philosophy in this book, it is only meant to highlight certain fundamental principles that are common among other Eastern philosophies as well, and are relevant to illustrate an important point in our discussion.

Human beings generally have varying degrees of three qualities, known in Sikh and Vedic philosophy as the stages of **Tamas, Rajas**, and **Satvik**. When a person is engrossed in the pursuit of worldly pleasures, and his mind is blinded by a range of uncontrolled emotions, such as anger, pride, selfishness, conceit, and jealousy, he is said to be in the **Tamas** state. When he is able to control the emotions but is driven mainly by ambition and desires in the pursuit of happiness, he is in the **Rajas** state. The stage of **Satvik** is achieved when he rises above the worldly desires and reaches a state of peace and tranquility in his being, and does not get engrossed in worldly affairs. The Sikh philosophy also believes in a fourth stage, which very few people achieve. This stage is known as **Sehaj,** the stage of intuitive poise. In this stage, the mind is centered and balanced, calm and at peace. This is where true understanding of the reality of life is obtained.

Disease only exists in the first three states of being (Tamas, Rajas, and Satvik); it does not exist in the fourth (Sehaj). It is important to understand that the way we live contributes to disease. When a person is engaged in worldly pursuits and experiences a range of emotions on a daily basis—from love, to anger, to hate, to jealousy—he attracts physical disease. In effect, disease occurs because of how we conduct ourselves in our life's pursuits. As such, headache is a symptom of an underlying cause that perhaps goes beyond the physical body.

It might be worthwhile to take a holistic approach toward preventing headaches by unifying the mind and body. This approach assesses all aspects of a patient's life: physical, mental, social, emotional, psychological, and spiritual. The best approach combines what ancient and modern traditions have to offer in a comprehensive treatment protocol. My aim is to integrate the modern scientific approach with the age-old wisdom of ancient traditions that preceded this Cartesian philosophy, and to provide solutions in headache management that utilize the best of what both have to offer. There are no quick fixes, and the patient is intimately involved in the decision-making process. The patient has equal responsibility for his or her own health, and has to have the right attitude. The "hey, Doc, fix me" attitude does not fit well with this type of integrative approach.

The optimal approach to the treatment of headache is in combining Western medicine with select alternative strategies that have proven to be effective. This is the approach taken in this book—to give insight into various healthcare systems that together will provide a unified cure to the common ailment of headache. The purpose of this book is for the readers to take charge of their own health and treat the cause of their headaches in a way that leads to optimal health and disease prevention.

The book is structured in five sections. I suggest you create a Freedom from Headache journal in which you write your notes and action steps as you complete the exercises suggested. This way you will better remember what you've read, your understanding will be deepened, and your motivation to apply the principles to obtain optimal health will be increased.

Section 1, Diagnosis of Headaches, introduces you to the basics of all headaches. Did you know that according to the International Headache Society, there are over 200 different types of headaches? This section will explore the most common headache types and their causes, and will attempt to explain how headaches develop.

Section 2, Conventional Treatment of Headache, discusses the conventional Western treatment strategies, including which drugs are available for which types of headaches, when to use medications for acute treatment, and when to use preventative ones. These questions are answered in a systematic manner, with the idea of helping you to understand the essential concepts that underlie why doctors choose different medications and treatments.

Section 3, Non-Pharmacologic Treatment of Headaches, explores the different holistic and natural approaches to headache treatment. We will discuss major concepts that underlie the wisdom of the age-old traditions such as acupuncture, homeopathy, yoga, and other treatment strategies.

Section 4, Special Situations, deals with specific groups of people who have unique characteristics and are susceptible to headaches in special ways.

Section 5, Stress and Headache Reduction Program, is the most important section, where I give you our philosophy on the treatment of headache, and our approach to dealing with any type of patient. The integrated approach takes the best of what conventional medicine has to offer, in terms of diagnosis and treatment, and combines it with the wisdom of ancient traditions.

Section I

DIAGNOSIS OF HEADACHES

CHAPTER 1
What Is a Headache Anyway?

- Headache is not a disease but a symptom of an underlying cause.
- Health is the optimal functioning of the body, mind, and soul.
- Physical health is just the outward representation of the health of the mind and soul.
- Headache is a biological disorder; it is not just "all in your head." It is a result of biochemical changes in the brain.
- Headache is not brain ache.

Do you suffer from headaches? Do you know someone, maybe even intimately, who suffers from headaches? Would you like to eliminate your headaches and lead a pain-free life? I presume that if you are reading this book, you have an interest in learning how to manage or even eliminate headaches. You might have an occasional headache or you might have a chronic condition. You might be a caregiver or a family member of someone who becomes incapacitated with migraine.

An Uncommon Dialogue

Let us have a conversation about headaches. Instead of being a passive reader, I want you to complete the action steps outlined at the end of each chapter so that we can help reduce your headaches. After all, if you don't take action, you will not achieve what you desire. In every decision, the mind battles with itself, to act or not to act, to do or not to do. We will be sharing a lot of information, but to get the most out of this book, you will need to act when action is required.

So, Do You Think You Are Healthy?

Headache does not occur in isolation. It is not a disease by itself but rather a symptom of some underlying cause. Headache is, more appropriately, an indication of the lack of health. To establish the right context, we need to define what we mean by health. Each individual is a triune being consisting of body, mind, and soul.

Health is the optimal functioning of this unity of body, mind, and soul rather than just an absence of disease. If a person is healthy physically but not mentally or spiritually, that person is not truly healthy and vice versa. In fact, **physical health is just the outward representation of the health of the mind and soul**. To be truly healthy throughout the various stages of life, one must know how to care for the health of the body, mind, and soul as intended by nature.

Applying this concept to headache management requires an understanding of what might be affecting the mind and spirit and thus causing the headache. It is possible that the cause of a particular headache is a medication side effect or muscle tension in the forehead from squinting in the sun too much. But if you suffer from chronic headaches, it is more likely that your headaches have an underlying cause that can be traced to your lifestyle. Even when there might be a genetic predisposition, such as in the case of migraine headaches, an underlying physical cause can be determined.

What Is a Headache?

Headache is a biological disorder resulting from biochemical changes in the brain. What causes these biochemical changes? The answer depends on who you ask. The International Headache Society (IHS) classifies headache in two broad categories, primary and secondary. According to IHS, primary headaches have no known cause while secondary headaches have an underlying organic pathology or disease.

Headache Is Not Brain Ache

A common misconception among people is that headaches are caused by some type of brain dysfunction. The brain does not cause headaches. In fact, if you were to cut a piece of the brain, there would be no pain. Yes, that is right! The brain itself has no pain receptors. The pain of headache comes from areas in the head that do have pain receptors. These include the coverings of the brain, known as the meninges, as well as the bones, the blood vessels, which wrap around and inside the brain, and the muscles of the face and head. According to conventional wisdom, inflammation and pressure on these receptors causes headache.

Are All Headaches the Same?

Again, this depends on the definition and the cause. If you define headaches based solely on symptoms, then there are over 150 different types of headaches. As you can see from the classification Chart A, the first distinction is to determine whether the headache is primary or secondary. It is important to note that this first distinction is based mainly on the symptoms. The cause is limited to whether there is an underlying organic cause, such as an aneurysm, tumor, or infection. In cases of primary headaches, the characteristics of the pain determine what type of headache it is: migraine, tension, or cluster.

Once your pain is placed in the appropriate category, it is subdivided

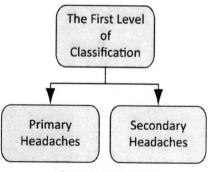

**Chart A: Primary/
Secondary Headaches**

into different types of primary and secondary headaches. A look at Chart B can give you an idea of how complex things can become as we go deeper into diagnostics. Even the classification itself can give you a headache. I call it classification-induced headache!

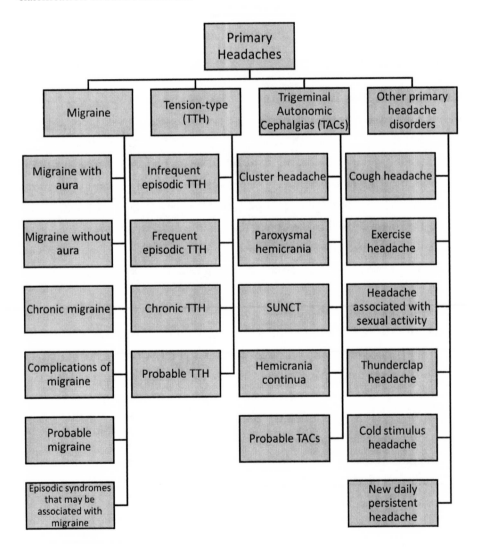

Chart B: Types of Primary Headaches

Most of the primary headaches belong to the first and second level classification. We will limit our discussions to those headaches. Some third-level headache suffers might also find solace in this book. Beyond that, it becomes too complicated to diagnose the headache, so it is advisable to consult a specialist.

Action Exercises

1. What in your opinion is the underlying cause of your headaches?
2. Do you feel you are healthy? If yes, what gives you this feeling? If not, what do you think you need to do to improve your personal health?

CHAPTER 2
Is Headache Common?

- You are not alone; headache is very common.
- The costs to the individual and society are enormous.
- Almost all headaches can be treated successfully.
- Migraine headaches in women usually decrease significantly over the age of forty-five.

Except for a handful of lucky people, headache happens to all of us. Headache does not discriminate; it happens to the best and the worst of us. Some people get headaches relatively infrequently and of a mild nature, while others suffer throughout their lives, curtailing the quality of their lives significantly. Almost every human being suffers from a headache at least once in his or her lifetime.

In this section, we will determine how common headache is, and we will examine the impact of headache on society. We will not spend a lot of time on this discussion, as we would like to get quickly to the cure of the headaches you have been suffering. However, it is helpful to put things in perspective and understand that you are not alone, and that almost everyone suffers from a headache at some point in their lives.

It is important to understand the incidence and prevalence of headache on a societal level.

Incidence refers to the percentage of the population who become headache sufferers on an annual basis. According to the International Headache Society (IHS), the incidence of both migraine-type and non-migraine-type headache is approximately 1 percent. That means one out of a hundred will suffer from headache every year.

Prevalence refers to the percentage of people who suffer from headaches at any given time. The graph summarizes the one-year prevalence of some common primary headache disorders. Let us look briefly at some interesting statistics:

1. By far, the most common headache disorder in the general population is episodic **tension-type headache (TTH)**, which affects approximately 40 percent of the population. (However, many headache specialists believe that a large number of migraine patients have been misclassified as TTH.)

2. **Episodic Migraine** is also a very common primary headache disorder affecting 18 percent of women and 6 to 7 percent of men.

3. In the United States, approximately thirty-six million people suffer from migraine headaches. It is a growing global epidemic. Worldwide, there are one billion migraine sufferers, and three billion suffer from TTH.

4. Approximately 10 percent of children suffer from migraine headaches, and it is equally prevalent in both sexes. The prevalence starts to increase in females as they transition from adolescence to mid-adulthood.

5. The presence of other medical conditions such as depression, anxiety, pain disorders, and stressful life events increase the likelihood of episodic migraine becoming chronic and thus harder to treat.

6. Every year, 95 percent of women and 90 percent of men experience at least one headache.

7. Chronic headaches occur for more than fifteen days per month and affect 5 percent of women and 2.8 percent of men.
8. According to the World Health Organization (WHO), migraine is the one of the world's most disabling disorders. It is the seventh most disabling disorder for women and the fourteenth most disabling for men.

It is important to realize that the prevalence of migraine-type headache sharply increases in the second decade of life. It levels off after that, and then starts to slowly decrease after the fourth or fifth decade, with the greatest decrease in women over the age of forty-five. It is important to note that it is most common in mid-life, when people are the most productive and busiest with their lives, going to school/work, earning a living, raising children, and participating in social activities.

What a Burdensome Problem

Chronic headaches can adversely affect the sufferers' quality of life because they are not able to participate in sports, social events, and entertainment activities. Headaches can also severely affect a person's career prospects.

Chronic headache adversely affects the productivity of a community. According to estimates, 51 percent of women and 38 percent of men with migraine headache miss the equivalent of six or more days of work per year. Frequent headaches increase the cost of medical care, which can be decreased by effective treatment and prevention. Chronic migraine produces more headache-related disability then episodic migraine.

We have to work together to improve the quality of life of our communities and ourselves. We can only do that by making everyone free of headaches by addressing the cause of the pain, while at the same time providing symptomatic relief. We will discuss this in more detail when we get to the chapters on treatment.

Migraine Is Under-Diagnosed

We can divide headache sufferers into different groups:

- Approximately one-third of patients have never seen a doctor for their headaches.
- A large segment of the headache sufferers have seen a doctor in the past but not recently. This segment used to be approximately 50 percent of all headache sufferers, but it has reduced to approximately 20 percent in recent years. From one perspective, this is good news, in that more people are going to a physician for treatment.
- About 47 percent of headache patients report that they have seen a physician recently.
- Fewer than 50 percent of patients with severe migraine headaches get help from professionals.
- Among those who go to a medical doctor, approximately two-thirds go to their primary providers, and only 16 percent see a specialist, such as a neurologist or a headache specialist.

In another survey, it was found that 71 percent of migraine sufferers said that they were dissatisfied with their usual acute treatments. The reasons for their dissatisfaction were:

- Pain relief takes too long (87 percent).
- Pain relief is incomplete (87 percent).
- The pain does not go away completely (85 percent).
- The medication doesn't always work (85 percent).
- The pain goes away and comes back (71 percent).
- Medications produce too many side effects (35 percent).

So you can see that you are not alone. Most patients are not satisfied with their current treatment strategies. The search for the optimal treatment continues.

You Are in Elite Company

Did you know that some famous people also suffered from severe headaches? Some of them were a cause of headaches themselves. The Roman emperor Julius Caesar suffered from severe headaches, as did Napoleon. Maybe the stress of writing the Declaration of Independence caused Thomas Jefferson's frequent headaches. As mentioned earlier, headache does not discriminate; in the American Civil War, the commanding generals Robert E. Lee and Ulysses S. Grant were both migraine sufferers. How headache affected the outcome of the war, we will leave to your speculation. Headache also influenced the writings of some famous authors, such as Lewis Carroll (author of *Alice in Wonderland*), Virginia Woolf, and Miguel de Cervantes. Painter Vincent Van Gogh suffered from headaches, and it is believed that the pain of migraine influenced at least some of his paintings. Some people believe that his unique style of painting and the use of vivid colors were influenced by the aura of migraine.

Seek and You Shall Find

The first issue is **awareness**, and the question to you is this: Are you seeking help for your headache? If you are not, the fact that you are reading this book is a step in the right direction. Another issue is whether you are doing something for the headache. If you are not being appropriately treated, then we need to improve therapy.

Our aim in this book is to promote awareness of the disease, the disability associated with it, and the various effective treatment options. For ongoing assessment, we need to define the goal of headache therapy to relieve pain and to restore your ability to function safely and with minimal side effects. However, the way we prioritize the various aspects of treatment varies from person to person, and it is therefore necessary to individualize treatment goals.

Action Exercises

1. How disabling is your headache? Has your quality of life diminished because of your headache?

2. How many physicians and alternative medical specialists have you consulted for treatment of your headaches? Write down the number of treatments you have been given, how long you tried each treatment, and how effective it was on a scale from 1 to 10.

3. Are you ready to experience headache relief?

4. Is there anything beneficial about your headaches?

CHAPTER 3
Headache Characteristics

- Headaches are diagnosed according to the characteristics of the pain.
- It is important to note the location of the pain, the type of pain, any exacerbating or relieving factors, what triggers the headache, the presence or absence of auras, and family history.
- Equally important are the factors that make you who you are: personality, likes/dislikes, the type of work you do, the level of stress you face on a daily basis and your ability to cope with it, and most importantly, your purpose in life.

L et us understand your headache. In order to do that, we are going to ask a few questions to identify the type of headache you are experiencing. This will determine the type of treatment recommended for you. It might be worthwhile to start writing the answers to these questions in your journal.

What Is the Flavor of Your Headache?

The first question you need to address is the **description** of the pain. Is it sharp, like a knife stabbing you in the head, or is it more like a toothache? Is it steady and constant, or is it throbbing, like a hammer hitting your head? Is it a pressure-type pain, or does it feel as if a rubber band is squeezing your head? Does your head feel as if it is going to explode? Sometimes people may have more than one type of pain. The pain can be mild one day and severe another day. It may be dull, achy, and all over the head one day, and throbbing, one-sided pain the next, with increased sensitivity to light and sound. Have you noticed more than one type of pain?

> **Migraine headache** is described as throbbing or pulsatile pain.
> **Tension-type headaches** are described as pressure-type, dull, achy, constant pain.
> **Cluster headaches** are severe and excruciating, and build to a crescendo within minutes.

Once you have determined the type of pain, the next question is the **location** of the pain. Is it on one side of the head or both sides? If it occurs on both sides of the head, do both sides hurt equally? Does it always occur on both sides, or is it sometimes unilateral (on one side)? Is one side more predominant? Is it in the front, in the forehead, or in the temples? Is it at the top of the head, also known as the vertex? Maybe it is in the back of the head just above the neck, or it is continuous with pain coming from the neck itself. The location can give a clue as to the type of headache it is. Also important is the duration of the pain. How long does it last?

Turn Off the Light, Please

After determining the type of pain and the location, the next question is whether there are any **exacerbating (worsening) factors**. In simple terms, these factors consistently bring on the pain or increase the intensity. These are called triggers. For example, some people notice worsening of the pain by bending forward. Others notice worsening of symptoms when sitting up from a lying-down position. Bright light or loud sounds may worsen the pain in some, while stress is an important trigger for most. What are your exacerbating factors, if any? Do you feel like locking yourself in a dark, quiet room so that no one disturbs you? Or do you get stressed out easily, which brings on the pain?

> **Migraine headaches** are unilateral, mainly in the temple region.
> **Tension-type headaches** are bilateral, mainly in the forehead or in the upper neck region.
> **Cluster headaches** are in and around one eye or cheek.

Typically, migraine headaches are triggered by certain internal or external factors. Some migraine sufferers are sensitive to foods such as chocolate, caffeine, cheese, and sugar, and other sufferers are sensitive to certain smells or changes in weather.

> **Migraine headaches** are triggered by many substances.
> **Tension-type headaches** are related to different types of stress.
> **Cluster headaches** have characteristic triggers, such as alcohol, nicotine, foods, and stress.

External triggers are substances in the external environment, exposure to which might result in headaches. Most triggers belong to this category. To cure headaches, these external triggers have to be individualized. For example, some migraineurs are allergic to chocolate. However, the chocolate we consume is a processed form of cacao beans that contains sugar, milk, and other substances. The sugar might be the cause and not the chocolate itself. We will discuss this in detail in the chapter on NAET.

Internal triggers are substances produced by the body, whether physiologically or pathologically, that may trigger a headache. The most commonly known are the hormonal changes that occur at the time of menstruation in some women. These women tend to have their headache predictably every month before, during, or after their menstrual period. There can be other internal triggers as well.

What Is That Burning, Rotting Smell?

The next most important question is whether there are any associated symptoms such as dizziness, blurred vision, vision loss in one or both eyes, or numbness or weakness in any part of the body. The question here is not whether you have *ever* had these symptoms. The question is whether your headache is **accompanied** by any of these symptoms.

Migraine can be accompanied by nausea, vomiting, dizziness, and sensitivity to light, sound, smells, and atmospheric pressure.

Of critical importance is the presence or absence of what are known as *focal neurological symptoms*. Any symptoms occurring in only one side of the body, such as weakness in the face, arm, or leg, can be due to some underlying process in the brain.

Do Not Disturb Me—I Am Taking a Nap

While it is important to note any causative or exacerbating factors, it is equally important to note what circumstances, activities, substances, and medications **relieve** the pain. If the headache is stress related, lying down and taking a nap might be helpful. Typically, in migraine patients, turning off the lights and lying down in a quiet, dark room minimizes the pain. It is important that you note your specific relieving factors.

Blame It on Your Parents

At this point, it is important to note that genes might also play a role in headaches. To ascertain the role of genetics, it is important to answer some key questions. Do any blood relatives have headaches? What are the characteristics of their headaches? At what age did you start experiencing your pain? Did the headaches start at a young age, or did they start later in life? Did you have episodes of unexplained abdominal pain and vomiting as a child? If you are older, did your headaches start after the age of fifty?

Watch Out, Here It Comes

In some cases, there might be an early warning sign of an oncoming headache. Known as *auras*, these typically precede the headache by minutes, hours, or even days. Do you have any warning signs before getting a headache? Do you become more sensitive to light or sound before you even feel the headache? Do you see any flickering or flashing lights, zigzag lines or blind spots, or experience any numbness or peculiar smells? If you get symptoms prior to the headache, can you describe the symptoms?

Many other factors can be very helpful in understanding the cause of headache and thus can aid in reaching a diagnosis: relationship to menstruation, seasonal changes, headaches occurring only in specific places, such as at work, in crowded places, or in air-conditioned rooms.

Who Are You?

Each person is unique in his or her personality, environment, attitudes, and circumstances. Understanding an individual is very helpful in devising non-pharmacologic treatment and prevention strategies. We suggest that you write your answers to the following questions:

1. What type of person are you? Are you an introvert or extrovert, talkative or quiet, sensitive or indifferent, a party type or a loner?
2. Are you a happy person?
3. Are you depressed? Do you worry a lot, or are you carefree?
4. What type of work do you do? Is your work physical, or do you sit in a chair all day?
5. Do you enjoy your work, or are you just passing the time? Are you working just to make enough money to pay the bills and put food on the table, or are you making a difference in people's lives? Do you have to work more than one job to make ends meet?
6. Do you take time out to relax?
7. Do you have fun? Do you have any hobbies or relaxing pastimes?
8. When was the last time you took a vacation? Was it a work vacation or a real vacation?

The following questions pertain to your relationships:

1. Are you married or single? If married, how is your family life?
2. Do you have a great relationship with your spouse or partner? Do you enjoy each other's company, or are you just putting up with each other? If it is not a happy marriage, how long has it been that way? Do you feel as if you are stuck in a loveless marriage with no hope for the future?
3. How is your relationship with your children? Are they a source of happiness or a major stress factor in your life?
4. Has life been unfair to you? Have you ever said or thought, *Why me?*

The following questions relate to your personality:

1. Do you stress easily? Are you a stressful person? In the chapter on stress management, we will ask you to take a short quiz to clarify your stress personality.
2. Do you get frustrated easily? Are you a controlling person, or do you like to delegate?
3. Do you get easily overwhelmed with circumstances?
4. Are you a leader or a follower?
5. Do you feel used up at the end of the day?

These may seem like a lot of questions, but it is important to understand your personality, your living and working environment, and the circumstances of your life to get to the true cause of your headaches. Identification of the source is half the treatment.

Let us illustrate a real life example here to clarify the discussions we have had so far.

JS is a twenty-eight-year-old who owns a fast-food store. He was referred for treatment of chronic headache in his forehead and the back of the neck, recurring for the past three to four years. For the past month, he had been experiencing pain in his temples, sometimes on one side, sometimes on the other. The headache was worsened with lack of sleep. He also experienced increased sensitivity to light and sound. During a particularly severe episode of throbbing pain, he had to go to the emergency room where he underwent extensive testing, including a lumbar puncture to check for infection or hemorrhage in the brain, but the tests showed that all was well with the brain.

He was prescribed narcotic medication and sent home. He continued to experience a similar type of headache every few days.

When he came to us, he was not actively having a headache but had been distressed because of the pain he had endured. His history was typical for migraine headache, and normally he would be considered for treatment with migraine-specific medications. However, further questioning revealed that he was a particularly stressful individual. He was in a family-owned business where there was pressure from his family members to make the business successful. He was recently married, but his wife was very supportive of him. He did not exercise regularly, and his diet was irregular. These discussions helped me decide to try lifestyle management techniques first before treating him with medication.

To start with, I gave him specific meditation exercises to help him relax. In addition, I advised that he start exercising, and I gave him specific dietary recommendations. He returned a month later feeling a little better. He had been exercising regularly, and had made some minor changes in his diet, which included eating breakfast regularly. He was meditating but not regularly. He had experienced two episodes of headache, which he attributed to dehydration. His energy level had improved, and he was generally feeling much better. Upon my reinforcement, he started meditating on a regular basis, and within a month, he noticed significant improvement. He noticed that when he did not get enough sleep and work became stressful, he got a headache. Now that he knew what to do, he could control his circumstances.

Thus, he was able to get control over his migraine headaches by implementing a program of lifestyle modification, dietary changes, regular exercise, stress management, and meditation. He realized that he needed to pursue his dreams, and some of the stress he had experienced was due to not following his life's purpose. He has now created a plan to do just that.

Action Exercises

1. Describe the characteristics of your headache.
2. Describe your characteristics as a person. What makes you who you are?

CHAPTER 4
Name That Headache

- All headaches are either primary (with no underlying identifiable cause) or secondary (due to an underlying medical problem).
- Majority of the secondary headaches have a benign, non-life-threatening cause.
- Life-threatening causes can be...well, life threatening, so you need to seek medical attention immediately.
- Learn the warning symptoms of potentially life-threatening causes of headaches.

So far, we have established that headache is, without question, one of the most common symptoms that neurologists evaluate. However, according to the International Headache Society (IHS), there are over 200 different headache types. We will briefly describe some of the more important types of headaches, such as migraine headaches, tension headaches, cluster headaches, sinus headaches, chronic headaches, rebound or medication-overuse headaches, and menstrual headaches. However, some headaches do not fit neatly into one specific category, which can complicate standard treatment strategies.

The symptoms of headaches vary from person to person, and each headache episode might have a different underlying reason. In other words, an individual may have attacks that range from mild to severe. It is conceivable that a person who suffers from migraine headaches might have some attacks that are so mild that they may not meet the diagnostic criteria for migraine headache. Finally, there may be a large overlap between the symptoms of migraine and tension-type headaches. This can sometimes lead to confusion about the correct diagnosis.

Classification of Headaches

In 1988, the IHS published a classification system for a broad range of headache disorders. These criteria for classification, which were based on an international consensus, were endorsed by the World Health Organization and incorporated into the International Classification of Diseases (ICD-10). The goal was to establish uniform terminology and consistent diagnostic criteria to serve as the basis of all conventional headache treatments. The criteria were revised in 2004, and are being revised again as the International Classification of Headache Disorders, 3rd edition. There are fourteen categories of headaches, with specific divisions and subdivisions within each category. Even the authors admit that the system is big and complicated, and not meant to be learned by heart. It was primarily introduced for clinical research.

Just because you have been diagnosed with a particular type of headache does not mean that you only suffer from that type of headache. It is important to note what type the majority of your headaches are. The classification is a tool, and should be used with care. You should never be locked in to a particular diagnosis.

What Category Are Your Headaches?

The IHS classification categorizes all headaches into two major groups: primary and secondary headaches.

- *Primary* headaches represent the vast majority of headaches treated in clinical practice. By definition, they are benign and not associated with any other disease.
- *Secondary* headaches are the result of some other underlying medical problem, such as a brain tumor, hemorrhage, infection, and a whole host of other benign and not so benign causes. The symptoms of secondary headaches represent a long list of underlying diseases. These headaches account for only 10 percent of headaches, but it is important for every headache specialist to ensure that a patient is not suffering from any of these underlying diseases.

The first job of a physician when evaluating a patient with a headache is to determine whether the headaches are primary or secondary. The cause or type of most headaches can be determined by a careful history and physical examination. It is especially critical to recognize the warning signals, which should raise red flags and prompt further testing. The focus of this book is to help prevent primary headaches.

Secondary Headache

Secondary headache is a headache with an identifiable cause. These causes can be divided into benign and life-threatening causes. Secondary headaches can lead to serious consequences because they result from an underlying disease. According to the IHS classification, there are eight different categories of secondary headaches. To educate our readers we have developed a list of benign and life-threatening causes of secondary headaches. These are just a small number of conditions for reference only. If you have symptoms of a secondary headache, we advise you to consult your doctor immediately.

Benign causes are not life threatening, and constitute more than 95 percent of all secondary headaches. There are many different causes of benign secondary headaches, which are listed below.

Allergies: A lot of you suffer from allergies. These can be due to known substances, such as peanuts, sugar, chocolate, caffeine, dust, pollen, and other allergens. Some of these allergies are manifested by headache, among other symptoms. Headaches associated with allergies are usually located in the forehead, between the eyes, or actually in the eye sockets, and are frequently accompanied by sneezing and runny nose, a condition known as *allergic rhinitis.*

Benign medical conditions causing secondary headaches

- Allergies
- Sinus problems
- Eyestrain
- Vision problems
- High blood pressure
- Temporomandibular joint (TMJ) syndrome
- Posttraumatic headaches
- Pseudotumor cerebri
- Cervical spine degenerative disc disease
- Medications
- Post-spinal tap

Sinusitis: The sinuses are air-filled cavities in the bones of the skull. Quite a lot of people are diagnosed with *sinus headache,* but for the majority of these patients, this is an erroneous diagnosis. Sinusitis refers to an infection of the sinuses, and can cause dull headaches on the area of the skull overlaying the particular sinuses. The most common locations for sinus headaches are the forehead, between the eyes, or over the cheeks. The pain is usually a steady ache that worsens with bending forward. It can radiate to the temples or other parts of the head. Fever is often present, and is usually accompanied by a thick, yellowish-green nasal discharge. The headaches may be accompanied by other symptoms of infection, such as nasal congestion, post-nasal drip, and facial tenderness over the area of the inflamed sinuses.

Sinus headaches may be mistaken for migraine headaches or TTH, especially when a person has chronic sinusitis. Standard treatment generally includes decongestants, or rarely, if the infection is due to a bacteria, antibiotics. Chronic sinusitis can be particularly difficult to treat with medications. Alternative treatments with acupuncture and NAET can be particularly helpful. In our opinion, sinus headaches are over-diagnosed, and patients take antibiotics all too readily without any clear indication of an infection, which can lead to secondary problems associated with antibiotic resistance.

TMJ syndrome: TMJ syndrome, as the name suggests, affects the **temporo-mandibular joint**. This is a hinge-like joint in front of your ear, between the jaw and the temple, where your lower jaw attaches to your skull. We use this joint more than most other joints in our bodies. Whenever you open your mouth for any reason, whether to chew, swallow, or talk, you use this joint. This joint can become inflamed or injured under certain conditions such as dental mal-alignment, gum disease, cavities, and even teeth clenching. In fact, there are only two reasons why this joint is injured: overuse and favoring one side of the mouth when chewing. Overuse occurs when people clench and grind their teeth. Some people grind their teeth at night, and are not even aware of it. Stress can cause this. Chewing on one side of the mouth can cause misalignment of the teeth over time, eventually causing pain in the TMJ. This pain may spread and cause a headache.

Treatment strategies for TMJ are numerous, including wearing a mouth guard, stress reduction, and medications. However, more than 90 percent of cases respond to simple measures aimed at improving your chewing habits and giving up chewing gum. If stress is an important cause, stress management is critical.

Life-threatening causes of secondary headache constitute a small minority of headaches. However, since they can be life threatening, it is important to recognize them and treat them appropriately. These conditions are listed in Appendix 1. Fortunately, these are relatively uncommon, but it is important to have a high index of suspicion as a precaution. While it is not your job to diagnose these conditions, it is your job to recognize when the headache is not just a headache, and if any of these symptoms are present, to avail yourself of the resources of your local emergency room or urgent care facility.

The next section lists the important symptoms you need to be aware of so that you can take action immediately if you have any of them. These symptoms are also known as the "red flags." Presence of any of these warrants an immediate and thorough investigation.

Warning symptoms of potentially life-threatening conditions:

- Headaches that reach a peak intensity in seconds to minutes, or sudden onset of the worst headache of your life
- Headaches triggered by coughing, bending over, sexual activity, or other physical exertion
- Headaches that begin or increase after trauma to the head or neck
- Focal neurologic symptoms such as speech difficulties, balance problems, visual changes, and numbness or weakness, especially on one side of the body
- Memory loss and/or confusion
- Onset of headaches after age forty
- Headaches that are not your usual type of headaches; i.e., there is a change in the pattern of underlying headache
- Abnormal neurologic examination, as performed by a physician
- Symptoms of other serious illness
- Headaches associated with neck stiffness
- Headaches associated with fever
- Headaches occurring for the first time in any patient, but especially in childhood or after the age of fifty

Warning! Stop! Call an Ambulance.

These potentially life-threatening situations need to be treated as an emergency.

I want to mention one such potentially life-threatening condition where the patient or a close witness has to initiate the notification of emergency services. Those patients who have a **sudden or abrupt headache that peaks in seconds**

or minutes (also known as Thunderclap Headache) require careful assessment to exclude potentially life-threatening causes such as subarachnoid hemorrhage (a type of bleeding in the brain), venous sinus thrombosis, arterial dissection, or raised intracranial pressure.

If these symptoms are noted and addressed, the chance of overlooking a sinister cause for headache is greatly diminished.

Action Exercises

1. Are your headaches primary or secondary?
2. Have you identified the potential cause of your headaches?

CHAPTER 5
Migraine Headaches

- There are four stages of migraine headache: prodrome, aura, pain of the headache, and the postdrome.
- There is no known cause of migraine, but it can be triggered by many substances.
- Migraine can be a very debilitating illness, causing untold suffering in migraineurs.
- Complicated migraine can be life threatening and is often associated with stroke, epilepsy, and other serious medical conditions.
- There is no reason to suffer in silence. There are many effective treatments for migraine.

Hippocrates, in 400 BC, described the visual aura of migraine preceding headache as "a shining light, usually in the right eye, followed by violent pain in the temple that eventually reaches the head and neck area."

Most of our patients have this to say about their headaches: "I just want to know what is causing my pain and how I can stop it."

According to the IHS classification, 2nd edition, there are three major types of primary headaches: migraine, tension-type (TTH), and cluster headaches. There is a fourth category of primary headaches, which constitutes headaches that do not fall into the three types listed above. In this chapter, we will focus on migraine headaches, as they can be particularly vexing and frustrating.

The distinction between migraine and TTH can sometimes be difficult because of their overlapping features. Migraine is a highly prevalent disorder, affecting up to 20 percent of the US population. It affects three times as many women as men and attacks people of every age and background. Before puberty, it affects both sexes equally, but after puberty, the incidence rises sharply in women. There is a genetic tendency as well; 70 to 90 percent of migraneurs have family members who suffer from migraine headaches. The headache intensity in migraine is, by definition, moderate to severe and often associated with other symptoms, such as nausea, vomiting, transient neurological symptoms, and disability. Most migraine headaches decrease in severity with age, although some patients' migraines worsen after menopause.

An Interesting Tidbit

Did you know that a migraine sufferer is known as a *migraineur*? However, in France, only a male migraine sufferer is called that. A female migraine sufferer is known as a *migraineuse*.

Symptoms of Migraine

There are six types of migraine headaches, but the most important distinction is between **migraine with aura** and **migraine without aura**. It is interesting to note that most patients with migraine can tell when they are going to have a headache. The headache is not generally the first symptom of the migraine. In fact, by the time the headache starts, the chemical changes that cause migraine have already begun minutes to hours before. Four stages have been described, although they vary greatly:

1. **Prodrome**: A lot of patients experience some symptoms prior to the onset of their headache. These are related to changes in the brain as the migraine begins. These prodromal symptoms can occur a few hours to a couple of days prior to the headache. Not everyone gets prodromal symptoms, and many patients do get them but are not aware of them. These can include mood changes, slurred speech, food cravings, fatigue, and yawning. Some patients crave chocolate as part of the prodrome. Sometimes family members may be the first to notice that the headache is coming because they notice the prodromal symptoms.

2. **Aura**: This is the second stage of the migraine. Auras can be visual, auditory, olfactory (sense of smell), and sensory, and they can affect the patient's speech. **Aura** (derived from the Greek word *aura*, which means *breath* or *gentle breeze*) refers to neurologic symptoms that develop slowly prior to the headache. Because aura is such a classic migraine phenomenon, its presence is nearly always diagnostic of this condition. However, only about one in eight people affected with migraine ever experiences an aura. Even with these people, auras tend to occur with some headaches but not all.

    In some patients, especially among the elderly, aura may be present without the headache. Because of this, it is important to differentiate between migraine and other disorders, such as transient cerebral ischemia, stroke, and seizures.

3. **Pain of the headache:** During an acute attack of migraine headache, you may have severe *throbbing pain*. It used to be thought that the throbbing was caused by dilation of the blood vessels supplying blood

to the brain. However, recent research studies into the mechanisms of the pain in migraine have found no correlation between the dilation of the blood vessels and the throbbing nature of the headache. The pain is usually *on one side of the head* and remains one-sided throughout the attack in most cases. Sometimes the pain can be on both sides or may radiate from one side to the other. Even when the pain is on both sides, one side is usually more painful than the other. Usually the pain lasts from hours to a day or so. On occasion, the pain may last longer. When the pain and the associated symptoms are unrelenting and last continuously for two or more days, it is known as **Status Migrainosus.**

The most common associated symptoms with the throbbing pain are *nausea, vomiting, sensitivity to light and sound, and worsening of the pain with physical activity*. Other less common symptoms are dizziness, lightheadedness, weakness, ringing in the ears, excessive sweating, visual difficulties, and sensitivity to smells. Some patients may also experience memory changes, mild confusion, and difficulty with concentration.

4. **Postdrome:** Once the pain of the headache and the other symptoms resolve, it is not necessarily the end of the migraine attack. A significant number of patients experience some symptoms that can last for hours to days. Many patients feel exhausted or drained, and may need to sleep for a few hours. Any symptom you experience before feeling well again is a postdrome.

Migraine Features

Table 1 describes the features of migraine headaches. Included are additional features of the migraine syndrome that are strongly supportive of the diagnosis. One of the most distinguishing features of migraine from other types of headache is its association with physical activity. This characteristic is specific for migraine headaches, which means that more than 95 percent of people with migraine have an increase in the intensity of their pain with any type of physical activity.

Table 1: Features of Migraine Headache

Common features

- More than five attacks lasting anywhere from four to seventy-two hours
- Unilateral (on one side of the head), but approximately 40 percent are bilateral
- Throbbing, but approximately half are non-pulsating
- Moderate-to-severe intensity
- Increase with physical exertion
- Associated symptoms of nausea, vomiting, sensitivity to light (photophobia), and sound (phonophobia), although vomiting is not as common.

Additional features

- Predictable timing around menstruation
- Stereotypical prodromal symptoms (symptoms that precede a headache). For example, you may experience visual symptoms such as flashing lights before the headache actually begins.
- Characteristic triggers
- Resolution of headache with sleep
- Family history
- Childhood precursors (motion sickness, episodic vomiting, or episodic vertigo)
- Osmophobia (sensitivity to smells)

Migraine Aura

The migraine aura is a complex array of symptoms that reflects *focal brain dysfunction*. The aura develops gradually over a five-to-twenty minute period, usually lasts for less than sixty minutes and is accompanied or followed by a headache. In some instances, particularly late in life, the aura may occur without an associated headache. Although the aura usually occurs before the headache in each attack, it may continue into the first several minutes of the headache or begin in the middle of an attack. The auras are most commonly visual and are often described as formless visual obscurations (described as heat waves rising off the road), bright silver, shining lights, or colorful fortification spectra.

Sensory aura is the second most common type of aura. Tingling may begin in one hand and over a period of minutes ascend the arm to the elbow and then jump to the same side of the face. Sometimes *mild weakness on one side of the body* may occur as a migraine aura, and sometimes, particularly in younger patients, *aphasia* (difficulty speaking or understanding speech) and/or *confusion* may usher in the headache. The neurologic symptoms are completely reversible.

Besides these two forms of migraine headache, there are many other less common types of migraine headaches and other primary headaches. Some of the more important ones are listed below.

Hemiplegic migraine: This migraine headache is a type of migraine with aura, and is associated with weakness and/or numbness of the arm or leg on the same side affected by the headache. The neurological symptoms may start before the headache or occur after the headache has already started. The symptoms usually disappear in a few hours, but on rare occasions, they can last longer or become permanent. The diagnosis of hemiplegic migraine should be entertained only after a thorough evaluation is performed by a trained physician to rule out any other underlying condition such as a brain tumor or stroke. There is a genetic basis for this condition, with mutations in certain genes, as there usually is a family history of it.

Retinal migraine (also known as **Ophthalmic migraine**): Retinal migraine affects vision. This type of headache usually presents as a temporary partial or total loss of vision in one eye, or not being able to see part of the visual field. Sometimes you may see twinkling lights called scintillations in one eye. The headache usually occurs during the visual symptoms, or may follow within sixty minutes. As you grow older, the visual symptoms may appear without the headache. Again, because this type of migraine can mimic other focal neurologic conditions, you should be evaluated by a specialist. The main difference between migraine with aura and retinal migraine is that the visual symptoms in retinal migraine occur in one eye only.

Basilar artery migraine: This is a potentially life-threatening migraine headache, but fortunately, it is very rare. It is a type of migraine with aura that affects the basilar artery, which is the main artery supplying blood to the area of the brain called the brainstem. The brainstem contains all the major centers that control the vital functions of the body, such as respiration and consciousness. This type of headache is accompanied by symptoms of severe dizziness, lack of coordination, double vision, slurred speech, and loss of consciousness. Some patients may have numbness and tingling around the lips and in their arms or legs. The symptoms usually precede the headache, and typically disappear when the headache starts, although they may continue for several days. The headache may radiate to the back of the neck, can be severe and throbbing, and is often associated with nausea and vomiting. This type of headache should not be treated with triptans or ergotamine. If you or someone you know has these symptoms, go immediately to the emergency room and be evaluated by an experienced physician.

Abdominal migraine: This is a chronic condition where patients may experience abdominal symptoms such as nausea, vomiting, diarrhea, and abdominal pain instead of the headache. These symptoms may occur with or without a headache, or may precede the headache, and usually occur in someone with a family history of headache. This is usually a diagnosis of exclusion, which means that other causes should be excluded first before making this diagnosis. This type of migraine tends to occur more commonly in children and is considered a childhood precursor of migraine. If a child is experiencing unexplained attacks of abdominal pain, consider abdominal migraine as a cause.

Migraine equivalent: Sometimes people experience all the signs and symptoms of migraine but without the headache. If you have episodes of abdominal pain of no apparent cause, nausea and/or vomiting, or other typical aura-like symptoms, but there is no headache, think migraine equivalent as a possibility. Abdominal symptoms without headache are more common in children. Older adults are also more prone to having migraine equivalents.

However, it is important to consider other more likely causes before labeling patients with this type of migraine.

Are Migraine Headaches Life Threatening?

Migraine headaches are not necessarily benign. In some cases, these headaches can induce several life-threatening conditions such as stroke, aneurysms, and coma, although they are exceedingly rare. There is also an increased association between migraines and seizures. However, migraine headaches are not fatal.

Common Migraine Myths

Myth #1: Migraine is just a really bad headache.

Reality: Migraine is a neurological disorder. The headache of migraine can be mild or severe. There is a genetic predisposition, and migraine patients have an unusual sensitivity to their internal and external environment. There are many associated physical reactions, and headache is just one of the symptoms.

Myth #2: Migraines are easily diagnosed.

Reality: Migraines are easily misdiagnosed. A majority of the migraineurs have never been properly diagnosed, so they never receive proper treatment.

Myth #3: Only women suffer from headaches.

Reality: Migraine does not discriminate. It affects people of both genders, all ages, and all races. However, it is more common in women by a 3:1 ratio.

Myth #4: If you do not have nausea or vomiting, then it's probably not a migraine.

Reality: Many patients never experience the accompanying symptoms of nausea or vomiting.

Myth #5: If you get headaches only with changes in the weather, they are probably not migraines and are more likely sinus headaches.

Reality: Changes in the weather can trigger migraines. Also, a runny nose or watery eyes are often part of the migraine itself.

Myth #6: *Only uptight, perfectionistic, Type-A personality people get migraines.*

Reality: There is no such thing as a migraine personality.

Myth #7: *Migraine is just an excuse to get off work.*

Reality: Tell that to a migraine sufferer and see what response you get. It is one of the most disabling conditions. Most migraine sufferers would gladly trade in their headaches for work.

Myth #8: *Children rarely get migraines.*

Reality: Migraine headache is common in children. Approximately 15 percent of teenagers suffer from migraine. Even children in grade school get migraines, although they are usually abdominal migraines.

Action Exercises

1. What are the characteristics of your pain? Are some of the features suggestive of migraine headaches?
2. Do you have any warning symptoms before the headaches begin? If so, what are they?
3. Do you have all the other symptoms but no headache?

CHAPTER 6

Migraine Triggers

- Any substance can be a potential trigger in susceptible individuals.
- MSG masquerades as many different things, so read the ingredients carefully.
- Most of the triggers can be cured using alternative strategies such as acupuncture, NAET, and homeopathy.
- Controlling or avoiding your triggers will help to lessen the burden of suffering from migraines.

People affected by migraine have what has been called a sensitive brain, and this sensitivity can be triggered by substances in the external and internal environment that start a whole cascade of events leading to the characteristic symptoms of a headache. This increased sensitivity is characterized by an enhanced response of the brain to specific sensory stimuli. However, in some cases, the response is not to a specific stimulus, but is a general over-excitation that exceeds the tolerance of an individual's body chemistry. In other words, the migraineur has increased sensitivity to both the *quality* and the *quantity* of sensory stimulation. Let us review some of the most common triggers and learn what you can do about them.

What Is a Trigger?

Simply put, *a trigger is a factor that increases the probability of a migraine attack.* It activates the mechanism in the brain that causes migraine. Unfortunately, you may not always realize what is setting off your headache. Triggers vary from person to person and from headache to headache. It is also possible that a specific trigger may lose its effectiveness as you grow older. Triggers do not cause headaches. They merely cause the sensitive brain to react a certain way, which leads to the headache. The exact mechanism by which the triggers cause headaches is not known.

There are certain caveats when it comes to triggers. A substance that triggers the brain of one patient may not cause any reaction in another patient. In other words, not everyone has the same triggers. Therefore, a list of potential triggers is worthwhile only as a starting point to see if a particular item may be a trigger for you. You have to make a list of triggers that cause your headaches. Having said that, let's examine some of the most common triggers.

It is important to remember that a particular trigger may not cause a headache every time. Patients have noticed a so-called threshold effect. You may have noticed it too. Some triggers may not trigger a headache individually, but if two or three triggers occur together and exceed your individual threshold, this may lead to a migraine attack. For example, skipping a meal may not trigger a headache, but skipping a meal *and* drinking wine *and* staying up late may trigger a headache, or skipping two meals in a row may trigger it.

Knowing your threshold is important. The threshold can be high or low. People who suffer from severe migraine headaches likely have a low threshold and are susceptible to even a minor exposure to the trigger.

Some triggers are related to your lifestyle. Abnormal sleep patterns, physical stress, eyestrain, and sexual activity are known triggers. So, let us focus on the most important triggers.

Stress

Stress is a very common trigger for migraine and TTH headaches. It can range from something as simple as eyestrain causing stress on the muscles of the eyes (oculomotor muscles) and muscles of the face, including the forehead and temples, to work-related stress causing severe migraines. The most likely stress is the one you experience in the daily grind: work, family responsibilities, disgruntled employees, deadlines, poor job satisfaction, and so on. In fact, stress itself is not bad; the level of satisfaction or dissatisfaction we get from the source of stress determines whether we feel the negative effects of it or reap the benefits. For example, I am experiencing stress as I am writing this book, but I am not stressed out, as the satisfaction of having written this book is reward enough. If you are constantly stressed out because of your circumstances and lack of satisfaction in your various endeavors, whether family, work, friends, or other relationships, this will lead to deterioration in your health. Headache is just one of the symptoms of unsatisfied stress.

The four close allies of stress, namely *frustration, anger, depression,* and *anxiety,* are all important emotional triggers. In modern society, we have become all too willing victims of the daily rat race, and these emotional triggers take a toll on our health. Lifestyle management and finding ways to decrease your personal stress are keys to achieving a headache-free existence.

Sleep Deprivation

People do not generally keep regular sleep hours. The lifestyle of the technology age and the fast pace of our society conspire to destroy our regular sleeping patterns. We either get too much or too little sleep. Both can cause headaches. People with migraine headache are particularly sensitive to irregularities in the sleep/wake cycle. If you do not adhere to a regular schedule, you will have an increased tendency to suffer from headaches. The reason for this is unknown, but it may have to do with the circadian rhythm. So, ensure that you get the amount of sleep your body needs at the right time.

There is no set amount per se, except it generally falls within five to eight hours per twenty-four-hour period. Every individual's needs are different. Some people cannot function on a minute less than eight hours, while some of us are bright-eyed and bushy-tailed after only five hours of sleep. Know yourself and get the amount you need. It has also been noted by sleep researchers that it is not enough to get the right amount of sleep; *when* you sleep can also be important. In other words, if you routinely sleep from 10:00 p.m. to 6:00 a.m., if one night you go to bed at midnight and wake up at 8:00 a.m., you may still get a migraine attack related to sleep. Try to go to bed and wake up at approximately the same time each day.

A majority of the people who suffer severe migraine have poor quality of sleep. In one study of people with transformed migraine, not one of the participants felt refreshed upon waking, and a majority of them woke up feeling tired. This can lead to the symptoms of chronic fatigue. For optimal treatment of the headache, addressing sleep issues is critical.

Excess Emotion

Excessive emotion and excitement can sometimes act as a trigger. This has been misinterpreted as a sign of weakness or an inability to handle stress, leading to the erroneous conclusion that migraine is a psychological disorder. In times past, this led to the stigma associated with migraine, causing people to hide their condition and suffer in silence. Migraine is not psychological; it is just another representation of the increased sensitivity of the brain to sensory stimulation.

Chocolate and Alcohol

I was given a mug at a hospital appreciation day, which has the saying, "Chocolate, the 5th food group" on it. I love chocolate. Lucky for me, I don't suffer from headaches. However, chocolate lovers with migraine headaches, beware! Quite a few migraine sufferers are sensitive to chocolate, which acts as a trigger. It is so common, in fact, that most avoidance diets for migraineurs list chocolate as one of the top items to eliminate from your diet. However, just because chocolate is a trigger for many patients does not mean that everyone is sensitive to it. If chocolate does not trigger your headache, you do not need to avoid it. Many migraine sufferers have no problem with chocolate. You may be sensitive to it, but by itself, it may not be enough to raise your sensitivity above the threshold.

It is unclear what exactly in chocolate triggers headaches. Is it the vasoactive amines that affect the blood vessels in the brain, or is it something else? Chocolate does contain phenylethylamine and caffeine, both of which have been found to trigger headaches. Phenylethylamine is also found in alcohol, and it is likely that this component of the alcohol is responsible for the alcohol-induced headache.

Chocolate that we eat contains not only the extract of the cacao bean but also milk, sugar, artificial flavors, emulsifiers, and other substances, such as nuts and raisins. Some people are sensitive to sugar, while others have a milk allergy, or lactose intolerance. Therefore, people with sensitivity to chocolate may have allergy to the cacao bean or to one or more of the other ingredients. It is your choice as to how to handle this trigger. Avoidance may be effective, especially if that has worked in the past. But if you want to get rid of the allergy so that it does not trigger the headache, you may want to try acupuncture, NAET, homeopathy, or another alternative strategy.

Dairy Products
Similar to chocolate, milk and dairy products can be triggers of headaches, and the problem is that they are not consumed by themselves; they are also part of the list of ingredients of many products, such as cookies, cakes, breads, and a whole host of other delectable food items. Avoiding dairy products completely may be difficult. (I can't imagine giving up ice cream altogether.) Alternative strategies such as those mentioned above are particularly useful for dairy products as well.

Cheese
Ah, pizza! It's the all-time American favorite, and what would pizza be without cheese? Cheese is another food item at the top of the list of migraine triggers. Tyramine is found in cheese, especially aged cheeses and cheddar cheese. It is thought that people with migraine are sensitive to tyramine-containing foods

because of a deficiency of an enzyme known as monoamine oxidase inhibitor (MAO) in their liver and blood, which is necessary to metabolize tyramine. Beer, wine, coffee, and yeast all contain tyramine, which may be the culprit causing headaches in migraine. As with other substances, you can either avoid foods containing cheese or utilize one of the effective alternative strategies to reduce your sensitivity to it.

Artificial Sweeteners

Artificial sweeteners that contain Aspartame, such as Nutrasweet, Equal, and Benevia, have been long recognized as triggers of headaches. Do you drink diet soda? If so, you are consuming aspartame, which has been linked to many neurological diseases, such as multiple sclerosis, brain cancers, arthritis, chronic fatigue syndrome, and epilepsy, among others. There is, however, no scientific data to support these links. More and more health care practitioners are advocating avoiding these artificial sweeteners and drinking clear water and fresh juices. If you are drinking diet soda to avoid gaining weight from the high-fructose corn syrup contained in regular soda, you need to know that aspartame actually stimulates appetite, so you are defeating your purpose. You are not doing yourself any favor by drinking diet soda. Any type of carbonated beverage is bad for your health and your headache.

MSG

MSG (monosodium glutamate) is a known potent trigger for migraine headaches. It is an artificial additive made through fermentation of corn, sugar beets, or sugar cane. It enhances the flavor of many foods. You may already know about the migraine-triggering effects of MSG, and you may be avoiding it conscientiously by checking the ingredients of packaged foods. Most processed foods contain MSG or its equivalents.

According to the website www.nomsg.com, MSG is now masquerading under different names. In the table below, we have provided a partial list for your benefit. As you can see from this list, if you thought you were safe by not buying products with MSG listed as one of the ingredients, you are sadly mistaken. You are still buying it, because it has so many pseudonyms. Is it any wonder that some people do not know why they are reacting to certain foods when they thought they were protecting themselves from their known trigger of MSG?

Definite sources of MSG include:

Autolyzed yeast, calcium caseinate, gelatin, hydrolyzed protein, sodium caseinate, yeast extract.

Possible sources of MSG include:

Textured protein, carrageenan, vegetable gum, seasonings, spices, flavorings, natural flavorings, chicken/beef/pork flavoring, smoke flavoring, bouillon, broth, stock, barley malt, malt extract, malt flavoring, whey protein, whey protein isolate/concentrate, soy protein, soy protein isolate, soy protein concentrate, soy sauce, soy extract

Other Dietary Triggers

A high-fat, high-sugar diet is an important diet-related trigger. There are other dietary triggers as well. These include caffeine, dehydration, prolonged hunger, and other less common triggers. Some of you who suffer from migraines may have noticed that if you do not eat foods at specific times, and you allow yourself to go hungry, this can trigger a migraine. **Prolonged hunger** creates relative hypoglycemia, so the body tends to burn fat, temporarily causing an increase in the amount of fat present in the blood. Hunger can also cause hormonal changes that can trigger the headache directly. **Dehydration** is another common trigger for headaches. This is vitally important since most people do not drink enough water. Lack of water increases the viscosity of blood, making it thicker, which results in platelet aggregation.

Caffeine is a potent vasoconstrictor, i.e., it causes blood vessels to constrict. Caffeine can be a headache reliever as well as a cause of headache. In small quantities, it has been shown to relieve headaches. As such, you can find caffeine in various painkillers. For people who do not drink coffee regularly, caffeine in the form of a cup of coffee might be helpful during an attack of headache. However, consuming caffeine consistently and in large quantities increases the level of fat in the blood and causes the aggregation of platelets, resulting in headache. In addition, since caffeine can be addictive, it can cause headaches due to its withdrawal effect. As few as three cups of coffee can be addictive, and stopping it suddenly can cause withdrawal headaches.

Nicotine found in cigarettes is a major trigger. **Perfumes** and other fragrances can be strong allergens for some individuals. This includes chemicals, paint fumes, and scented soaps and detergents. Natural **environmental factors** such as changes in weather patterns, damp, cloudy weather, heat, and humidity have all been linked to headaches. Artificial environmental factors such as pollution, dust, pollen, and motor vehicle exhaust can also precipitate headaches.

There are many more possible triggers than what we have listed here. In fact, any substance can be a trigger in a susceptible individual. You have to ascertain the particular triggers that apply to you.

If chocolate is a trigger for you, then definitely you should avoid chocolate and limit its intake. However, if it is not, and you love chocolate, there is no reason to deprive yourself of indulging in it occasionally. We do not believe in lists of forbidden foods unless you make such a list after determining your particular triggers.

For some of you, the only defense is to go back to basics and live a life of purity—purity of body, mind, and soul. As a general principle, the more natural foods we eat, the healthier we are. The principles of health as propounded by the ancient sages are still the best. The more technologically advanced we become, the more triggers we create, and the more we suffer from headaches.

More so than the actual substances that can act as triggers, what we have found is the most important trigger for patients with migraine is a lack of pattern, or lack of a schedule. Most migraine patients do well with a certain routine. For example, people find that sleeping the same amount and at the same time every night, eating at the same time every day, or exercising the same amount every day is very helpful.

Disrupting this pattern by staying up late one night or skipping a meal can lead to a headache. If you want to incorporate something new, make it a daily habit rather than shocking your system with it. If something out of the ordinary is going to happen, such as a trip, or a wedding, or a night out on the town, you need to take steps prior to the event to minimize the deleterious effects.

Action Exercises

1. Do you know what *your* triggers are, if any?

2. If not, keep a headache diary. Examine some of the common factors. What did you eat, drink, and do? Where did you go before you experienced the headache? Can you correlate the headaches to any particular triggers?

3. Do you get stressed out easily? Is your headache more frequent when you are stressed?

4. Do you get headaches at the end of the pay period?

CHAPTER 7

Other Conditions Associated with Migraine

- People with migraine have an increased risk of depression, and vice versa.
- There is also a correlation between migraine and seizures.
- Too little, too much, or poor quality of sleep, all have an impact on migraine.
- Up to one third of persons with stroke will have a history of migraine, even if there is no other link between these two conditions.
- Certain features are common to both stroke and migraine.
- Migraine may be a risk factor for stroke in women who take birth control pills and who smoke.

A s you may have realized, people with migraine have an increased sensitivity to change in their environment, whether it is internal or external. In fact, this sensitivity is the hallmark of migraine. Effective treatment of migraine requires an adequate understanding and recognition of this increased sensitivity. This is not limited to the nerve cells; other cells in the body also reflect this enhanced responsiveness to the environment. Therefore, it is common to see evidence of other conditions or diseases in patients with migraine headaches.

Comorbidity is a situation where one or more diseases coexist more often than would be expected if the occurrence of each disease were by random chance, but where one condition is not the cause of the other(s). For example, patients with migraine tend to have other co-existing conditions such as depression, epilepsy, stroke, irritable bowel syndrome (IBS), fibromyalgia (FBM), chronic fatigue syndrome (CFS), premenstrual syndrome (PMS), anxiety, insomnia and other sleep disturbances, and bipolar disorder. One of the reasons it is important to recognize these comorbidities is that they may have important implications in the treatment of your headaches. In this chapter, we will discuss some of these comorbidities.

Migraine and Stroke: A Coincidence?

Migraine has been linked to stroke in a variety of ways. Both these disorders are common; therefore, it is not unusual for both conditions to coexist in the same person. In some instances, migraine can *cause* a stroke, and in others, it can be a *risk factor* for stroke. Certain underlying conditions predispose to both migraine and stroke. Let us explore some of these associations in more detail.

Stroke is the third leading cause of death, affecting two out of a thousand persons per year.

Given the high prevalence of migraine in the general population, up to one third of persons with stroke will have a history of migraine, even if there is no other link between these two conditions. Usually the patients who experience stroke associated with a migraine headache tend to be younger than age forty-five. In fact, 27 percent of all strokes in patients under the age of forty-five are preceded by a severe migraine headache.

Common Symptoms

Certain symptoms are common to both stroke and migraine. In order to understand this concept, it will be helpful to first define stroke. A stroke is to the brain what heart attack is to the heart. Stroke is characterized by lack of blood flow to a part of the brain. This occurs when a blood vessel that carries oxygen and nutrients to the brain bursts or is blocked by a clot. When that occurs, the part of the brain that does not get the blood (and thus the oxygen) dies. A transient ischemic attack (TIA, also known as a minor stroke) has the same symptoms as stroke, except that the symptoms resolve completely within a short period, usually minutes to hours. **Migraine with aura** has certain focal features that can be confused with symptoms of a stroke or, more commonly, TIA.

The less common varieties of migraine, such as hemiplegic migraine, retinal migraine, basilar migraine, and migraine with prolonged aura can be particularly difficult to differentiate from stroke. The opposite can occur as well; a stroke can be mistaken for a migraine, especially when the stroke is associated with a headache.

Migrainous infarction is a rare condition in which a stroke occurs *during* a migraine attack. It occurs more commonly in women in their thirties, especially those who smoke, because the arteries of smokers tend to be constricted. During a migraine attack, there is further narrowing of the arteries, which, if severe enough, can compromise blood flow to the affected area of the brain, causing a stroke. Fortunately, migrainous infarction does not occur very frequently.

Migraine Is a Risk Factor for Stroke

Migraine is now thought to be an independent risk factor for stroke, just as high blood pressure, high cholesterol, and diabetes are. This is especially true for women, although men are also at a slightly higher risk, especially those younger than forty-five years of age. Many studies conducted not only in the United States but in France, Italy, and Denmark have shown this association. Migraine with aura seems to present a higher risk than migraine without aura. The use of contraceptive pills has also been associated with stroke, especially the ones containing higher doses of estrogen. The highest risk appears to be in women with migraine who use contraceptive pills containing estrogen and who are smokers. However, keep in mind that even though the risk is increased compared to women who do not have migraine, the absolute risk is still relatively small.

Implications for Treatment

The first step toward reducing the risk of stroke is to identify those who have a high risk. Managing risk factors (high blood pressure, high cholesterol, smoking) is critical for decreasing the risk of stroke. Migraineurs should be cognizant of their risk factors and avoid smoking and using contraceptive pills, especially those containing high doses of estrogen.

The American Heart Association, along with other organizations, has developed guidelines for assessing cardiovascular risk. These include lifestyle modifications to reduce this risk and managing risk factors such as high cholesterol, high blood pressure, diabetes, and obesity. These organizations have developed an atherosclerotic cardiovascular disease (ASCVD) risk estimator to estimate the ten-year and lifetime risk for ASCVD. If you are interested in learning your risk of stroke, you should ask your physician to help you by applying the ASCVD risk estimator. This is especially important if your physician may be prescribing some common medications for your migraine such as triptans, ergots, or DHE, as these drugs may have cardiovascular side effects, and should not be used by persons who have a high risk of stroke.

Depression

The link between depression and migraine has been studied extensively. Each disease predisposes to the other. In other words, people with migraine have an increased risk of depression, and vice versa. The correlation between these two conditions may be as high as 50 percent. It has also been found that a majority of the people (more than 60 percent) who suffer from mild depression and migraine tend to receive little or no treatment for their migraine. Similarly, many people are not being treated effectively for their depression, as it is believed to result from their headache. Both migraine and depression are progressive conditions, which means they increase in frequency and severity with age. If not treated properly early on, both diseases can become more difficult to treat. Therefore, it is vitally important to diagnose and treat depression and migraine early on to prevent higher levels of severity later. If the underlying cause of both conditions (and other comorbidities as well) is not addressed properly, patients will continue to suffer. In addition, migraine patients suffering from depression and anxiety have a higher risk of developing increased severity of their migraine as well as medication-overuse headaches.

Epilepsy

There is also a correlation between migraine and seizures. Epilepsy, the tendency to have repeated seizures, is due to abnormal excitation of the cells of the brain. There also appears to be a genetic predisposition for both conditions, especially when they coexist. People with one condition are twice as likely to have the other. The strongest association exists in migraine with aura. However, this comorbidity is not recognized, most likely because the seriousness of epilepsy may foreshadow the migraine. Sometimes, the differentiation between the two conditions may be difficult, as the symptoms of migraine can mimic those of epilepsy. In some cases, the patients with epilepsy may not report their migraines, as their preventative medication (which may be an epilepsy medication) may be controlling their headaches. This may become important if the medication is changed to another anti-epileptic medication, which may not be as effective for migraine. The reverse is also true.

Sleep Disturbances

Too little, too much, or poor quality of sleep all have an impact on migraine, but this relationship is variable. The cause for both poor quality of sleep and migraine can be the same, which in the majority of cases is stress. In migraine patients who have chronic insomnia, addressing the insomnia is very important, as lack of sleep exacerbates the headache. If not treated, this can lead to the symptoms of chronic fatigue. If you wake up with a migraine, it may indicate a problem with your sleep. If you are not sleeping well, or if you are getting too little or too much sleep, all these can trigger your headache.

Action Exercises

1. Are you a migraineur who also suffers from depression?
2. How good is your sleep? Do you have difficulty falling asleep or staying asleep? Do you wake up refreshed?
3. Are you a young woman who smokes and takes birth control pills?

CHAPTER 8

Tension-Type Headaches (TTH) and Other Primary Headaches

- TTHs are very common and usually are not incapacitating.
- Most TTHs occur during periods of high stress or emotion.
- Taking medications too frequently can lead to the development of rebound headaches, where the treatment becomes the culprit.
- Medication-overuse headache is an example of our society's addiction to instant gratification.
- If you are suffering from frequent headaches, it is time to get expert help.

Although tension-type headache (TTH) is the most frequent of the primary headaches, it is the least distinct and least understood of the headache disorders. In fact, its clinical diagnosis is based chiefly on the absence of symptoms that characterize migraine. In many cases, patients are suffering from migraine, but have been erroneously diagnosed as having TTH headaches. Most people will get a TTH at least once in their life, and approximately 90 percent will experience it more than once. There are no significant risk factors, but the most common causes are fatigue and stress. Most people with this type of pain do not seek professional help, since these headaches usually are not disabling and do not interfere significantly with daily routines unless they become more frequent.

Most people with TTH state that the headaches usually occur during or after times of high emotion, such as anger, anxiety, fear, stress, and irritability. They also occur with chronic depression. Typically, the headaches occur on both sides of the head (bilateral). The pain is usually pressure-type, steady, non-pulsating, dull, and persistent, and is usually not worsened with exertion or physical activity. The intensity of the pain is typically mild to moderate. These headaches may be accompanied by tightness in the muscles of the neck and shoulders. People usually describe the pain as a vise-like or squeezing type of pain. Rarely is there sensitivity to light and sound.

There are two types of TTH:

- **Episodic TTH:** These headaches are brief, lasting minutes to hours, and typically occur fewer than fifteen days per month. These are further subdivided into **Frequent** and **Infrequent Episodic TTH.**
- **Chronic TTH:** Chronic headaches occur at least fifteen days per month for at least six months. These are also called chronic daily headaches. We will discuss them in detail shortly.

Other causes of TTH:

- Fever
- Eyestrain
- Insomnia
- Depression
- Poor posture

- Sinus problems and allergies
- Caffeine withdrawal
- Environmental factors
- Cervical muscle spasm (neck pain)

Let us see if you suffer from TTH. Analyze the characteristics outlined below and see if they fit your headache.

Characteristics of TTH:

- Mild to moderate pain
- Headache occurs on both sides of the head, in the forehead, in the back of the head, or all over the head.
- Pain does not awaken you at night.
- Pain is not worsened with physical activity.
- There is no aura or premonitory symptoms.
- Pain is pressure-like, steady, dull, achy, and constant.
- There is no associated nausea and/or vomiting.
- There may be sensitivity to light or sound, but not to both.

As with migraine headaches, there are other types of TTH. In fact, some of the causes of TTH may result in a migraine or TTH. For example, *caffeine withdrawal* can cause both migraine and TTH. Although the term *triggers* usually refers to migraine headaches, we can think of these as TTH triggers. Some *environmental factors*, such as pollution, exhaust fumes, colognes and perfumes, and chemicals may cause TTH in patients who are not susceptible to migraine headaches.

Treatment of TTH

Treatment of TTH is divided into non-pharmacologic and pharmacologic. At this time, we will briefly mention the optimal approach to TTH. Indeed, you should utilize these non-pharmacologic strategies before resorting to strong medications. Since TTH, as the name suggests, are due to some type of tension, stress, or underlying negative emotion, you should try to address the cause. It is not enough to address the symptoms by taking analgesics. If the headaches are becoming more frequent, it is imperative that you identify the possible causes and eliminate them. Stress management is particularly effective in relieving stress-induced headaches. Obtaining adequate sleep, exercising regularly, relaxing, and meditating are very effective measures that obviate the need for pharmacologic therapy in most cases.

Medication Overuse Headache (MOH)

There is another type of headache known as medication over use headache (MOH), which used to be known as *rebound headache*. This headache is not part of the above classification of primary and secondary headaches. This headache is due to excessive use of medications, whether they are over-the-counter or prescription medications. MOH occurs primarily in patients with an underlying headache disorder. It is one of the most difficult problems associated with analgesic medications. It is associated with even the simplest of these types of painkillers. Medication overuse headache is an example of a vicious cycle that is very difficult to break. Typically, patients start using medications for very frequent headaches. As they take more and more medications for their headaches, their bodies become dependent on the medications and develop tolerance to them, a process called *central sensitization*. Therefore, they need to take more of the medications to get the same pain relief. Eventually, they reach a stage where the medication itself causes the headache. They enter into a vicious cycle where they cannot stop taking the medication.

Medication overuse headache is one of the biggest problems that headache and particularly migraine patients face. Every headache sufferer should become familiar with this type of headache. According to IHS, it is "the most common cause of migraine headache occurring on more than fifteen days per month, and of a mixed picture of migraine-type and TTH on more than fifteen days per month."

There is a phenomenon known to many migraine sufferers called *tachyphylaxis*, which means the medication becomes less effective over time as the body gets used to it. Patients have to take an increasingly higher dose to achieve the same relief. This causes the brain to produce pain when it is time for the medicine. This is the cause of MOH. Most patients with chronic daily headaches (CDH) require almost daily use of pain medication. These MOH are usually superimposed on their regular migraine headaches.

Rebound or MOH is a perfect example of our society's addiction to instant gratification. Patients want quick relief from their headache without seeking a cure for the cause of the pain. Since the cause is not addressed properly, the headache keeps recurring. The patient keeps taking medication to get quick relief, and as the pain-free period between headaches lessens, the patient becomes more dependent on the medication, leading to the vicious cycle where the cure becomes the cause of further pain and suffering. This is true for both OTC medications and stronger prescription medications, as we shall see in the section on medications. In fact, it has been shown that all drugs used for the treatment of headache can cause MOH.

In addition, frequent use of these medications can lower the threshold for headache so that patients develop increased sensitivity to the triggers that bring on headaches. This adds to the vicious cycle, and the patient, instead of becoming headache free, now has an additional problem of medication dependency.

The only way to treat MOH is to stop the medication, which is not an easy task. We will discuss the treatment of MOH in the chapter on chronic daily headaches.

Other Primary Headaches
Some of the less common types of primary headaches include:

Primary exertional headache:
The headaches of exertional migraine are brought on almost exclusively by physical exertion. This is more commonly seen in children, and it usually occurs in combination with other triggers, such as fatigue. This type of headache is more common in hot and humid weather, and likely results from overheating of the body, which acts as the trigger for the migraine.

Primary headache associated with sexual activity (used to be called coital headache or benign sex headache):
This relatively rare cause of headache occurs more commonly in adults, and as the name suggests, is brought on by sexual activity. It occurs abruptly during

orgasm. This type of headache should be distinguished from a more serious, potentially life-threatening underlying secondary cause, namely subarachnoid hemorrhage. This more serious type of headache occurs due to sudden rupture of a blood vessel in the brain, likely due to increased blood pressure inside the skull. If a person with no prior history of headache during sex develops a sudden severe headache, the so-called "worst headache of my life," the cause might be brain hemorrhage, which can be life threatening.

Caffeine withdrawal headache:
Caffeine is a drug, and as with any habit-forming drug, you can develop a dependency on it. People who have become used to drinking a caffeinated beverage on a regular basis can experience headaches if they reduce its consumption or stop it altogether. This type of headache can range from mild to severe, and can be accompanied by other symptoms of withdrawal, such as anxiety, nausea, and irritability.

Hypnic headache:
This type of headache mainly affects elderly patients. The pain is usually throbbing in character, and it wakes patients from sleep. The pain can be unilateral or bilateral. There is usually no associated sensitivity to light or sound, no nausea or vomiting, or any other neurological symptoms. Hypnic headache usually responds well to a medication called lithium, although verapamil and indomethacin have also been found to be helpful.

Action Exercises

1. Are you a stressful person? What causes your stress?
2. Can you relate your TTH occurrence with feeling stressed out? How frequent is your TTH?
3. Is there something you can do to lessen the cause of your tension-related headaches?

CHAPTER 9
Cluster Headaches

- Cluster headaches predominantly affect men.
- Cluster headaches occur in clusters of intense pain almost daily for a period of one to two months.
- The pain of the headache can be severe and excruciating.
- The most effective treatment of cluster headaches is inhalation of 100 percent oxygen.
- Administration of lidocaine in the nostrils is also an effective treatment for this type of headache.

Cluster headaches are a type of vascular headache affecting nearly two million people in the United States. It is an unusual condition as it is likely to affect six times more men than women. Women who have cluster headaches tend to have somewhat masculine features. Although far less common than either TTH or migraine headaches, people with cluster headaches can be easily recognized during a painful event. These headaches are cyclic in nature and come in clusters, hence the name. In 90 percent of the people who suffer cluster headaches, the attacks of pain usually occur in cycles that last four to eight weeks followed by a pain-free period. Attacks of pain tend to recur at the same hour each day for the duration of the cluster bout. However, after the susceptible period has passed, the person does not experience any further symptoms until the next cluster. During the cluster period, the headaches can wax and wane over a period of days, weeks, and sometimes months. In rare situations, they can occur continuously for years. For that unfortunate person, it really is a headache from hell.

Characteristics of the Pain

The pain of cluster headaches is described as one of the worst pains ever experienced. It starts quickly, without warning, and reaches a crescendo within fifteen minutes. It is deep, non-fluctuating, and explosive in quality. In addition, 10 to 20 percent of patients can have paroxysms of stabbing, icepick-like pain around the eye that lasts for a few seconds. The symptoms resolve in one to two minutes. This pain is usually described very eloquently by patients: "It feels like a hot poker pushing into my eye," or "It feels like someone is stabbing my eye with a sharp knife." The pain is always on one side, and generally affects the same side in subsequent bouts. Typically, this type of headache may cause you to awaken suddenly from the pain.

Pseudonyms of cluster headache:
- Migrainous neuralgia
- Horton's headache
- Atypical facial neuralgia
- Sphenopalatine neuralgia
- Raeder's Syndrome
- Histamine neuralgia

As opposed to migraine headache, where the pain is exacerbated with physical activity and movement, cluster headache patients often hit their heads against the wall or inflict pain on other areas of the body to distract their attention from the severe pain of the headache. Migraine patients prefer to lie still in a dark, quiet room.

Signs and Symptoms

The majority of cluster headache sufferers report some or all of the following symptoms, all of which are unilateral:

1. Severe, sharp, stabbing pain around the orbit of the eye or the temple
2. Tearing and redness in the eyes (lacrimation and conjunctival injection)
3. Droopy eyelid (ptosis)
4. Stuffy nose and drainage of clear fluid from one nostril (rhinorrhea)
5. Sweating on the forehead, abdomen, and trunk
6. Flushed face

As you can see from the description of the symptoms, the pain characteristics are much different from migraine headaches. Typically, in cluster there is usually no nausea or vomiting.

Precipitating Factors

Approximately 50 percent of people who suffer cluster headaches report increased sensitivity to alcohol during a cluster bout. People who are sensitive to alcohol note that attacks are triggered within forty-five minutes after the ingestion of modest amounts of alcohol. Some people report other precipitating factors, including stress, exposure to heat or cold, glare, hay fever attacks, and occasionally, specific foods (chocolate, eggs, dairy products). There is some evidence that head trauma can precipitate the syndrome as well.

Like migraine, cluster headaches are vascular; however, the exact mechanisms behind the severe pain and the symptoms are not known. Many theories have been postulated, including alterations in the serotonin levels, same as in migraine. According to another theory, because of the seasonal correlations of cluster headaches, there must be a relationship with the patient's biological clock, the *circadian rhythm*. The exact nature of the relationship is not clear.

Circadian Rhythm

A circadian rhythm is an internal twenty-four-hour cycle, our own body clock. It is derived from the Latin word *circa*, which means *around*, and *diem*, which means *day—about a day*. It depends on external cues such as sunlight and temperature. It determines our sleeping and feeding patterns, and is linked to the daylight and darkness cycle. Brain wave activity and hormone production are linked to this cycle. This circadian clock in humans is located in the *suprachiasmatic nucleus (SCN)*, a group of cells in the hypothalamus. The retina transmits information about the length of the day to the SCN, which sends it to the pineal gland where the hormone melatonin is secreted in response to darkness. (Melatonin secretion peaks at night.) Cluster headaches have been linked to disruption of the circadian rhythm.

Acute Treatment

Acute treatment is designed to treat the patient during the cluster bout until the bout is over. Since the pain is so excruciating, people are more likely to be compliant with their treatment if the right remedy can be found. Fortunately, most people know when their cluster is going to start and end. The treatment strategy is no different from treating migraine headache: acute therapy for the pain and preventative therapy to reduce the recurrence and severity of the episodes. Since the attacks are brief and peak rapidly, oral medications are generally not very effective because they are absorbed slowly by the body, whereas inhalational medications bring quicker relief.

The best treatment for acute pain relief in the majority of cluster headache sufferers is the inhalation of 100 percent oxygen via a tight-fitting mask at a flow rate of eight to ten liters per minute for ten to fifteen minutes. This treatment can dramatically reduce the intensity of the pain in about 80 percent of patients. This mode of therapy has recently been substantiated by controlled studies. Oxygen inhalations may be repeated up to five times per day. The exact mechanism by which oxygen treats the headache is not clear, although oxygen stimulates the synthesis of serotonin in the central nervous system (CNS).

Another specific treatment for cluster headaches is the intranasal administration of lidocaine. Although no controlled clinical trials of lidocaine have been conducted, anecdotal evidence suggests that approximately 60 percent of patients can respond to this therapy. One milliliter of 4 percent lidocaine is administered into the nostril on the same side as the pain. Relief can occur in as little as five minutes.

Both ergotamine (in aerosol form) and dihydroergotamine (DHE) injection (intravenous) are very effective in stopping acute attacks. However, the DHE intravenous can only be given in a hospital setting, so other therapies are tried before resorting to a trip to the emergency room. Sumatriptan and the other triptans such as zolmitriptan have also been found to have varying degrees of success in treating acute cluster headaches, especially the non-oral forms of these medications.

Treatment of Cluster Headache:
- Inhalation of 100 percent oxygen
- Intranasal lidocaine 4 percent
- Ergotamine (inhaled)
- DHE (intravenous)
- Sumatriptan
- Other triptans

Preventative Therapy

The major prophylactic drugs for the cluster syndrome are prednisone, lithium, methysergide, and ergotamine. Lithium appears to be particularly effective for the chronic form of the disorder. A combination of verapamil (a beta-blocker) with either valproate, topiramate, or lithium is particularly effective in preventing cluster headaches.

SUNCT Headache

There is another type of vascular headache known as SUNCT headache. This stands for Short lasting, Unilateral, Neuralgiform headache with Conjunctival injection and Tearing. As you can see, the features are very similar to cluster headaches. They also affect men more than women, are more common over the age of fifty, last for seconds to minutes, and usually occur during the day. However, patients may have many attacks per hour. Fortunately, these types of headaches are very rare. The treatment does differ from cluster headaches, as these are treated with antiepileptic drugs or steroids and NOT with oxygen.

Action Exercises

1. If you think you suffer from cluster headaches, describe your symptoms.
2. Do you have any other circadian rhythm problems?
3. How is your sleep? Do you get fatigued easily?

CHAPTER 10
Laboratory Testing

- Laboratory testing is not routinely performed in the evaluation of a patient suffering regular headaches.
- The routine use of imaging procedures is not warranted in patients with migraine or TTH when there has been no recent change in the pattern of the headache, no history of seizures, and/or no focal neurological findings.
- Tests are usually performed when there is a high suspicion of a secondary cause of the headaches.

L aboratory testing is not routinely performed in the evaluation of a headache patient. No test can diagnose the different headache types. The main reason for performing laboratory testing is to determine the presence of a secondary headache disorder. We have included this chapter in this book so that you can become familiar with the different tests in case you have to go to the ER and one of these tests is performed, or your doctor orders one.

Common Tests

Blood Tests:

These include the **complete blood count** (CBC) which measures the various components of blood, including white blood cells (WBCs), red blood cells (RBCs), and platelets. The **chemistry panels** evaluates the levels of different chemicals in the blood, including glucose (blood sugar), electrolytes such as sodium and potassium, liver enzymes, and tests for kidney function. Some abnormalities in these chemicals can point to conditions that can cause recurrent headaches. Tests of **thyroid function** can diagnose either hypo- or hyperthyroidism, either of which can cause headaches. Sometimes measuring the levels of different vitamins can uncover deficiencies of these vitamins. Magnesium levels can also be checked. In addition, some medications prescribed for headaches may cause side effects such as lowering the numbers of white blood cells and platelets. We can also measure the levels of certain medications in the blood.

Computerized Axial Tomography (CAT or simply CT) Scan:

This test obtains three-dimensional (3D) images of the head using X-rays. It is normally used to detect underlying structural brain abnormalities such as hemorrhage, tumors, or infection. It is particularly useful in the emergent evaluation of a headache patient in whom a brain hemorrhage is suspected. For other conditions, the MRI is more sensitive and has a better resolution. (MRI gives us better 3D images.) In some cases, an iodine-based dye is injected into the bloodstream while a CT is performed in order to provide better information about the brain. Some people are allergic to the dye, however.

Magnetic Resonance Imaging (MRI):

This test also obtains 3D images of the brain but uses magnetic waves instead of X-rays. It creates images that are generally superior in quality to those created by a CT scan. The limitation of the MRI is that since it utilizes a magnetic field produced by a strong magnet, you cannot undergo MRI if you have any metal implants such as pacemakers, metal braces or plates, orthopedic screws, as these can degrade the quality of the images and may cause harm to you and/or damage the magnet. Another limitation of the MRI is that the patient is placed in a cylindrical tunnel, which may cause claustrophobia in some. A type of MRI known as **magnetic resonance angiography (MRA)** utilizes magnetic waves to assess the flow of blood inside and outside the brain. An MRA looks for such conditions as aneurysms, stenoses (narrowing of the arteries), vascular malformations (congenital abnormalities of the arteries and veins), and other vascular conditions.

The main purpose of an MRI is to rule out the possibility of an underlying structural cause, such as a tumor, aneurysm, stroke, or infection. The MRI does not tell you anything about the headache itself.

Cerebral Angiogram:

An angiogram is an invasive test where dye is injected into the arteries, such as the carotid arteries in the neck, outlines them, and sequential pictures are taken. This helps in evaluating the layout of the arteries in order to map their course and assess any abnormalities.

Lumbar Puncture (LP):

An LP, also known as a spinal tap, is performed in cases of suspected brain infection, tumor, or hemorrhage, or other less common conditions. It involves inserting a needle into the middle of the lower back to remove spinal fluid for analysis or to relieve pressure in the brain. It is not performed routinely in the evaluation of a patient with headache, but in some instances of severe headaches, it is a very important test.

Positron Emission Tomography (PET):

This scan is not routinely used in the evaluation of patients with headache. It measures the brain's structure, activity, and the pattern of blood flow.

Scientific studies have shown that advanced imaging techniques, such as CT and MRI, have helped in the diagnosis of only 0.18 percent (less than two per

1000) of patients. In two studies of imaging in patients with TTH, no significant lesions were detected at all. In people whose headaches were not classified, the rate of finding a significant lesion was slightly more than 1 percent.

The American Academy of Neurology has therefore concluded that CT and MRI are not likely to uncover significant neurological diseases as a cause of the headaches. Thus, the routine use of these procedures is not warranted in people whose headaches fit the definition of recurrent migraine or TTH, who have had no recent change in headache pattern, have no history of seizures, and no focal neurological findings.

In this imaging-friendly world, this may be a little disconcerting for some people. This is an instance where the diagnosis and the treatment is based mainly upon clinical data, i.e., on your description of your headaches and the physical and neurological examination. Therefore, it is crucial that the history be as accurate as possible.

The utility of these tests becomes important in cases where your physician suspects there may be a secondary cause of your headaches. For example, if a brain tumor, hemorrhage, infections such as meningitis or encephalitis, seizures, or allergies are suspected, appropriate tests can be performed to evaluate such possibilities. These tests are advisable for patients who have the red flag warning signs we mentioned earlier, or who have an atypical (unexpected) presentation of their headache.

CHAPTER 11
What Causes Headaches?

- A deficiency in serotonin, a brain chemical, is implicated in the origin of migraine headaches.
- Migraine patients have a genetic susceptibility.
- Unless a certain threshold of susceptibility is reached, the symptoms of migraine do not develop.
- Headache is generally felt in the area supplied by the trigeminal nerve.

According to conventional wisdom, primary headaches have no known cause. When we talk about the cause, we are concerned about the processes that take place at the cellular level. If you were to study the history of headache treatments, you would be amazed at the types of beliefs about the causes of headaches, especially migraine headaches, as well as the treatments that various cultures and civilizations have utilized to cure their headaches. Probable causes have ranged from possession by malevolent beings, evil spirits, demons, and other supernatural phenomenon, to punishment for sin, to the vascular theory, to the neurovascular theory, and finally to the activation of the trigemino-cervical pain system. Let us explore the current understanding about the origins of this complex disorder.

If you recall, the core features of migraine headaches are throbbing pain, often on one side of the head, accompanied by nausea and sensitivity to light, sound, and head movement. Because of the throbbing nature of the pain, migraine is also known as a *vascular* disorder (related to the circulation of the blood). However, this is not entirely true as up to one-third of migraine sufferers do not have throbbing pain, and modern imaging has demonstrated that the vascular changes are not linked to the pain of migraine.

Trigemino-Vascular Theory

In short, the current theory regarding the genesis of migraine is that it is a combination of genetics and environmental factors, which activate the trigeminal system. This is known as the *trigemino-vascular theory*. Headache is usually felt mainly in the distribution of the trigeminal nerve (the major nerve of the face and head) and some of the upper cervical spinal roots. This implies that there is unrestrained firing of cells in the spinal trigeminal nucleus. Specific areas in the brain influence the incoming pain pathways and blood flow to the specific parts of the brain responsible for the pain; these areas are the aminergic areas in the periaqueductal gray matter and locus coeruleus. Instability in the pain control system means that there is a continuous discharge when there is stimulation from higher centers of the brain (cortex, hypothalamus) due to stress or by excessive input from the special senses (senses of smell, vision, hearing, taste and touch). In essence, migraine is the result of instability in this pain control system.

Serotonin

The brain chemical *serotonin* is one of the main culprits of migraine. Quite often, there is an insufficient amount of serotonin in the brains of migraine patients, or the receptors to which it binds are less sensitive to it, which makes it lose its effectiveness in sending messages from one part of the brain to another. Serotonin has also been implicated in other important functions of the brain, including feeding behaviors, temperature regulation, sexual behavior, and sleep. It also has a role in controlling depression and anxiety. As we will see later, medications have been developed to act directly on serotonin systems, or to mimic serotonin to control the symptoms of migraine. Many theories have been postulated as to how serotonin causes headaches. It is thought that serotonin can have the following effects:

- Release of serotonin from platelets can trigger the headaches.
- Release of serotonin from certain nerve fibers results in an acute attack.
- Changes in the metabolism of serotonin induce an attack.

The frequency of migraine attacks vary from once in a lifetime to almost daily, which indicates that there is variability in the degree of predisposition to migraine. There is a threshold of susceptibility, which means that even though there is a genetic susceptibility, unless a certain threshold is reached, the person will not experience migraine even in the presence of triggers. To understand migraine, we need to consider both the factors that influence the threshold of a person's susceptibility to a migraine attack and how an attack is triggered.

Genetic Susceptibility and Brain Sensitivity

Migraine is more common in patients who have a family history of it. Because of this genetic basis, people with migraine have inherited the so-called migrainous genes. This means they have what can be called a sensitive brain. The current thinking is that there is an underlying instability in the pain-processing systems of people affected by migraine causing them to be overly sensitive to environmental changes. This is seen as a heightened sensitivity to various stimuli such as bright light, sounds, smells, and even touch. About 25 percent of patients experience certain symptoms in the hours prior to the start of their headache, including yawning, irritability, hunger, and mood change. These premonitory symptoms are thought to originate in the part of the brain known as the hypothalamus. Episodes may recur regularly as if initiated by some type of internal clock located in the hypothalamus.

Relationship of Diet to Headache

The presence of obesity has been associated with more severe and frequent migraine attacks. This has been attributed to the fact that this condition is known to cause inflammatory changes in the blood and blood vessels. In a recent scientific study, it was found that obese patients had a higher proportion of severe headache attacks compared to patients who were not obese. Obese and morbidly obese people had increased frequency and severity of headache as well as increased sensitivity to light and sound.

As we have learned, the brain chemical serotonin is involved in the production of headaches. Serotonin levels are affected by the presence of vitamin B6. Vitamin B6 is required for production of an amino acid known as tryptophan, which is a building block of serotonin. Low levels of B6 decrease the production of tryptophan, resulting in low levels of serotonin. B6 and tryptophan are present in many fruits, vegetables, and grains.

The majority of the serotonin in the body (over 90 percent) is contained in a type of cells in the blood called platelets. These platelets play an integral role in the formation of blood clots. Under normal circumstances, platelets flow smoothly in the blood. When they become activated, these platelets aggregate (cluster together). It is still unknown what causes platelets to aggregate in migraine patients. Aggregation of the platelets releases serotonin (among other substances). The initial high level of serotonin released is followed by a rapid decrease as the serotonin is broken down. This in part is responsible for the symptoms of migraine.

It is believed that one of the factors causing increased platelet aggregation is the increase in the levels of certain fatty substances in the blood. These fatty substances are blood lipids, which include cholesterol and triglycerides as well as other fatty acids. Adding extra fat to the blood makes the blood thicker, as the fat globules take up more space, displacing other constituents. This makes it easier for the platelets to aggregate.

A study evaluating the effects of diet in migraine conducted at Loma Linda University in California showed that lowering the amount of fats in the blood (by changing dietary consumption of fat) allowed the platelets to function properly, thereby reducing the release of serotonin.

Almost all known triggers of migraine also cause an elevation of blood fat levels.

According to current thinking, the genesis of migraine headache is a complex process. In a susceptible individual, one who has the genetic predisposition to having migraines, the process starts with a dysregulation of the level of certain neurons in the hypothalamus, brainstem, and the cortex. This creates a wave of electrophysiologic hyperactivity followed by suppression of brain activity known as **cortical spreading depression (CSD)**. This activates the trigemino-cevical complex (an area known as the periaqueductal gray), the thalamus, and the sensory cortex, all of which are pain pathways, by possibly releasing a chemical known as **cacitonin gene-related peptide** (CGRP) as well as other factors. This activates and sensitizes different parts of the brain, which results in the production of the associated symptoms of light and sound sensitivity, nausea, dizziness, and fatigue. Activation of the pain pathways triggers the production of the headache.

There is currently an intense interest in the CGRP. This chemical has been identified in the blood during a migraine attack. Furthermore, infusing this chemical triggers a migraine, and some experimental CGRP receptor antagonists (blockers) have been shown to stop a migraine attack. Will this be an effective treatment for migraine? Only time and further research will tell.

According to some migraine researchers at UCLA, while we still don't fully understand what causes migraine headache, what has become clear is that during a migraine attack, there is a storm of electrical and chemical activity that "switches on" different areas of the brain and surrounding nerves to cause the symptoms of migraine. The goal of treatment is to "switch off" these abnormally activated brain regions and nerves.

CONVENTIONAL
TREATMENT
OF HEADACHE

CHAPTER 12
Basics of Treatment

Now that we have established a basic understanding of headaches, it is time to put it all together to see what we can do about your pain and suffering. There are many headache treatments, including conventional medical treatments as well as alternative therapies. It is ironic that treatments that have been successfully in use for hundreds if not thousands of years such as herbal treatments, acupuncture, ayurvedic treatments, and lifestyle changes have been termed alternative, while modern medical treatments, which have been in vogue for not even a century, are considered conventional or traditional, when it should be the other way around.

When we talk about **secondary** headaches, the conventional treatments are concerned with treating the **underlying cause** of the headache, such as infection or tumor in the brain. For **primary** headache disorders, most conventional treatment is aimed at **symptomatic** relief (pain control), and does not address the cause of the pain. Many drugs address the symptoms of the pain as well as the associated symptoms of anxiety, insomnia, depression, mood changes, and the like. There is no perfect treatment for headache. But this statement is true only for conventional medicine. The conventional assumption that there is no *identifiable* cause does not mean that there is *no* cause. It just means that our current diagnostic acumen is not able to identify the cause. According to medical textbooks, headaches, especially migraines, are chronic conditions that cannot be prevented or cured, but can be *managed* only by our current approaches. Alternative medicine can provide help in diagnosing the causes and recommending a cure.

As we know in the case of migraine, the symptoms are due to the brain's increased sensitivity to sensory stimuli. This can be addressed in many different ways. In cases where excess emotion triggers a headache, a patient might prefer to hide the condition, as in many cultures it is considered a sign of weakness to succumb to emotions. However, this results in suppressing the very nature of your true self, your self-esteem, your vitality. This is equally dangerous, as it will eventually lead to serious health problems. By avoiding the vicissitudes of life, you avoid experiencing the joy of living. Optimal treatment strategy includes understanding emotion and its role in causing the headaches. You are not completely healthy until you are healthy in body, mind, and spirit. It is important to note that living entails full self-expression.

If you curtail the expression of your true self and are continually limiting your activities so that you are not able to express yourself fully, you are not truly healthy.

This leads us to the optimal approach to true headache freedom: combining medical treatment with natural and alternative methods. The two approaches complement each other.

Before we get into that, let us discuss some of the conventional approaches. As practitioners of Integrative Medicine, a field that combines the best of both modern technological and alternative approaches, we would be remiss in our duty if we did not address the conventional medical approaches, because these treatments do have a role in the optimal treatment of a patient if used judiciously. According to this approach, the mainstay of treating migraine and TTH is medications. A vast majority of the patients who see a physician for their headache will be prescribed some type of medication, whether over-the-counter

(OTC) pain relievers or prescription medications. Using medications carefully can be extremely effective in relieving suffering.

All people suffering from migraine need acute relief. Some of you may even need medications for prevention of your headaches, especially those of you suffering from chronic repeated headaches. Let us examine each of these conventional approaches.

CHAPTER 13
Tips to Stop the Pain of Headache

When you are in excruciating pain from a headache, all you can think about is getting rid of it. Instead of reaching for that pill or injection, however, there are certain non-medication treatments you can try on yourself to eliminate the pain. Not all of these will necessarily work for you, but you may be pleasantly surprised at the effectiveness of at least some of them. We will discuss these non-pharmacological treatments in more detail, but here we will give you some tips to reduce the pain of the headache.

Eleven ways to stop migraine at home without taking medications:

1. **Ice**: One effective method is to put a cold compress such as an ice pack on the base of the skull or to the forehead. Most of you will find that ice is a very good form of pain relief in acute headaches. Cold constricts the blood vessels, limiting the flow of blood to the head. It overrides the pain messages to the brain and lowers muscle contraction by lowering your metabolism. If you are using an ice pack, make sure there is a

barrier between the ice pack and the skin, such as a towel. The sooner you apply the ice pack after the pain starts, the faster and more complete the pain relief will be.

2. **Massage therapy**: Massage your face, especially your temples. You may consider dipping your fingers in cold water while massaging your temples and the back of your neck. Get someone to massage your neck and upper shoulders. This combines the soothing effect of massage with the constricting effect of blood vessels described in #1.

3. **Exercise**: While migraine headache can be worsened with physical activity, some people find aerobic exercise in the early stages of the headache to be helpful in decreasing the pain.

4. **Acupressure**: Massage the fleshy web between the thumb and the index finger of the hand for quick relief. This is an important acupressure point for headache relief. Using the opposite hand, squeeze the flesh with your thumb on one side and one or more fingers on the other side. Massage using a rhythmic squeezing action for one to two minutes. Switch hands and do it as long as necessary. Don't squeeze so hard as to cause pain, but hard enough to feel the squeeze.

5. **Relaxation**: Close your eyes and take a few deep breaths to slow your brain wave activity. Lie down in a quiet, dark room, avoiding bright or flashing lights. Turn off the television and all electronic devices such as laptops, tablets, mobile phones, and desktop computers.

6. **Water**: Make sure you are properly hydrated. Not drinking enough water can cause dehydration-induced headache. Drink a glass of cold water or a nutritious beverage such as natural juice. Water is the real elixir of life.

7. **Laughter**: We have all heard that laughter is the best medicine. Laughter is one of the best methods for quickly relieving stress. It can be particularly effective in relieving headache triggered by stress. Try watching a light-hearted comedy while relaxing in a comfortable chair.

8. **Sex**: Another method of obtaining quick relief is sexual activity. Instead of invoking the popular excuse, "Not tonight honey, I have a headache," use headache as an excuse to engage in sexual activity.

9. **Aromatherapy**: Do not underestimate the effectiveness of aromatherapy. You can rub **peppermint oil** on your temples, especially for tension headaches. This method is said to be as effective as taking a NSAID for pain relief. Other oils used for headache relief include **lavender** and **chamomile**. Inhaling the oils can be deeply relaxing. **Eucalyptus oil**, alone or in combination with **clove oil, camphor,** and **caraway,** has been shown to be very effective in controlling headache.

10. **Ginger and aloe**: These are ancient Ayurvedic remedies. Drinking ginger tea can be helpful in some patients with headache. For others, aloe juice can create a cooling effect.

11. **Specific breathing exercises**: Proper breathing techniques are very effective in relieving headaches. For acute pain relief, a simple breathing exercise can be very helpful. Close the right nostril with the thumb of the right hand. Inhale deeply through the left nostril. At the end of the inhalation, close the left nostril with the middle finger of the right hand, and let go of the right nostril. Exhale completely through the right nostril. Then inhale through the same nostril, taking a long deep breath. At the end of the inhalation, close the right nostril with the thumb again, while letting go of the left nostril. Repeat this **alternate nostril breathing technique** twenty-five times.

CHAPTER 14
Conventional Approach to Headache Treatment: Acute Treatment

- Effective conventional therapies for acute pain relief of migraine include OTC and prescription medications including nonspecific and migraine-specific medications.
- Triptans are the most effective migraine-specific medications for acute pain relief.
- Opioids and other narcotic medications should be used sparingly, as they can cause tolerance and addiction.
- There are established guidelines for the use of medications for relief of the headache of migraine.

W hen you are suffering from an acute headache, you need quick relief. If the natural methods discussed in the previous chapter do not provide relief, it is important to examine other options to control the pain. Pragmatic medical approach divides the treatment of recurrent headaches into *acute* treatment and *prophylactic* or *preventative* treatment.

Acute Treatment

Acute treatment includes all the strategies utilized to treat the acute pain including over-the-counter (OTC) medications and prescription medications.

The current general principles of acute migraine care include the following:

1. **Treat the headache as early as possible** to reduce the intensity and duration of the pain as well as the accompanying features. Waiting until the headache becomes moderate-to-severe seems to decrease the effectiveness of acute treatments.

2. **Individualize the treatment** to both the individual and the type of the pain. Instead of using the step approach (discussed on the next page), use the most effective therapy early. The step approach may increase the pain, disability, and impact of the headache.

3. **Use the correct dose and formulation** specific for the particular type of headache. This means using the stratified approach, not only in terms of choosing the right medication, but also the right dosage of the medication. In other words, it is more effective to start with the right dose than to start with a low dose and slowly increase it until you get the desired effect.

4. **The route of administration** is especially important in patients experiencing severe nausea and vomiting. In these cases, the tablet form of the medication may not be effective, and the patient may need an alternative mode of administration, such as an injection, nasal spray, or tablets that dissolve in the mouth.

5. Generally, the use of acute medication should be restricted to a maximum of two to three days per week to avoid rebound or medication-overuse headache.

6. Everyone needs acute treatment.

When choosing acute therapy, several factors need to be taken into consideration:

1. What is the **time of onset** of headache and the resulting severity? In other words, when and how quickly does the headache come on? In situations where you have very rapid onset of headache, non-oral medications should be considered for more immediate symptom relief.

2. Consider the **symptom profile**. If you are experiencing significant nausea and vomiting, consider use of non-oral agents or anti-emetics (medications used for nausea and/or vomiting).

3. **Frequent headaches could be the result of medication overuse.** In this situation, you need to take extra caution when taking a prescription medication.

4. Finally, when selecting therapy, take into consideration your **experience with treatments in the past**, both the successes and failures, as well as treatment preferences.

Early treatment can often lead to more complete relief and reduced headache recurrence. The intensity of the treatment program should be matched to the severity of the disease. When the triptans are not effective in reducing the pain of the migraine headache, this could be an indication that other nonspecific agents, including NSAIDs, combination analgesics, opioids, and neuroleptics, might not be effective as well.

Step Care vs. Stratified Care

There are two strategies for initial therapy:

Step care is the use of medications in a sequential order, starting with the lowest level of treatment, independent of the characteristics of the attack. This approach to treatment is not necessarily based on the individual needs of the patient. In this approach, the patient's treatment is started with low-dose OTC medications such as acetaminophen or ibuprofen. If your headache does not go away, your doctor may prescribe stronger medications such as a higher dose of ibuprofen or weak narcotics. If your headache is still recalcitrant to treatment, the next step is to prescribe stronger opioids or triptans.

Stratified care is treatment based on attack characteristics, including intensity and severity of the headache, associated symptoms, and disability. This strategy is individually tailored to specific patient needs. Stratified care takes into account patient preferences for treatment and allows the patient to select medications for each particular attack. This gives more control to the patient in deciding which medication works best.

Stratified care is advantageous because it is more likely to be effective in reducing pain and disability and improving overall patient satisfaction. It also has the potential to provide improved cost-effective care through fewer visits to the doctor's office and fewer failed prescriptions. However, even with an ideal stratified care plan, treatment of an individual attack may fail and require backup or rescue medication.

OTC Medications

Most headache sufferers have tried some form of OTC medication before seeing a physician. In fact, most headache sufferers do not seek professional help on a regular basis. A multitude of medications can be found on the shelves of major pharmacies and drug stores. Be aware that most medications have two names, the brand name and the generic name. For the same generic medication, there may be many brand names. These drugs are non-specific and designed to provide temporary relief of acute pain. Despite the large number of medications with different brand names available on the market, the ingredients in most of these medications are mainly three: *aspirin*, *acetaminophen*, and *ibuprofen*.

The major differences in OTC medications are the amount of the generic medication and the combination with other medications. For example, Extra Strength Excedrin is a combination of aspirin, acetaminophen, and caffeine. Similarly, Advil is the brand name for ibuprofen. Other brand names for ibuprofen are Nuprin, Motrin, and Medipren. Appendix 2 lists some of the more commonly available OTC medications, their uses, and common side effects.

One of the important points to note from the table is that there is no substantial difference between the various brands. For example, Extra Strength Excedrin and Excedrin Migraine are substantially the same products targeted to different market segments.

There is clear evidence of benefit for these medications in the treatment of headache. The ones that have strong scientific evidence in the treatment of migraine headaches include aspirin, aspirin plus caffeine (brand name Anacin), aspirin plus caffeine plus acetaminophen (brand name Excedrin), ibuprofen, and naproxen. A recent study showed that the combination medications (such as Excedrin) were more effective than single medications for treatment of TTH.

The other important point is that OTC medications are not without potential side effects. Just because they are available without a prescription does not mean they cannot cause serious side effects. The most commonly seen problem with aspirin and ibuprofen (which belongs to the class of medications called non-steroidal anti-inflammatory drugs, or NSAIDS) is irritation of the gastro-intestinal system (stomach and intestines). In rare instances, this can be potentially serious leading to life-threatening bleeding in the gut. As with any medications, the more effective they are, the more likely they are to have side effects. Even acetaminophen, which is generally thought to be one of the safer medications, can cause long-term complications such as liver or kidney damage if used too frequently. A word of caution: any medication, whether OTC or not, should be used with discretion. In addition, too frequent use of these medications can lead to medication-overuse headaches.

Prescription Medications

When OTC medications fail to relieve the pain, most headache sufferers will end up in a doctor's office to seek stronger prescription medications.

In order for any prescription to work, the most critical factor at this stage is that physicians discuss all the possible behavioral modifications that are typically quite successful in treating headaches with a minimum of medications.

Before prescribing migraine-specific medications, a physician may first try non-specific medications including stronger NSAIDs. It is important to realize that all these medications can have side effects. Some of the common side effects are listed in the table, but in rare cases, there could be some serious side effects. In addition, some medications, especially the narcotics, lose their effectiveness over time, and have tremendous addictive properties. Over time, people can develop tolerance and dependence on these medications. In some cases, this might cause rebound headaches. Appendix 3 lists some of the non-specific medications commonly used for the treatment of acute headaches.

Scientific studies have shown three non-specific medications to be effective in managing migraine headaches. Two of these, prochlorperazine (brand name Compazine) and chlorpromazine (brand name Thorazine) are given intravenously, so they are generally reserved for the emergency room. The one medication that can be used outside of the ER is butorphanol (brand name Stadol), which is generally used as a nasal spray. It is also a narcotic, specifically an opioid, and should be used with caution. However, it is an effective non-specific medication in the treatment of migraine headaches.

Another drug that is less commonly used these days but is still an effective medication is isometheptine (brand name Midrin).

Migraine-Specific Medications

All of these specific medications have a common effect of interacting with the neurotransmitter serotonin in the brain. This chemical has many important roles in our brain including preventing headaches. These drugs either act like serotonin or have similar effects, such as reducing the inflammation and causing the arteries and veins to constrict, thereby reducing blood flow to specific parts of the brain.

Triptans

Most of these migraine-specific drugs belong to a group of medications called **triptans**. The more technical term for triptans is selective serotonin receptor agonists. The important non-triptan drugs are dihydroergotamine (DHE) and ergotamine (Cafergot, Ergostat).

The advent of triptans was a very important step in the acute treatment of migraine. The first triptan synthesized was sumatriptan in 1984. Triptans are not typical pain medications as we traditionally think of them. It may be useful to think of migraine headache as a cascade of events (a domino-type effect, if you will); once the symptoms start, the headache follows a predictable course. Triptans have an abortive effect, which, according to our analogy, can be thought of as stopping the cascade of events before the cascade has gone too far. The advent of triptans changed the way headaches were treated.

At the time of this writing, seven triptans are in general use in the United States as abortive therapy for migraines. These are available in a number of formulations. For better response, it is important to match the formulation to the headache characteristics and the patient's preferences. Appendix 4 lists the triptans in common use in the United States. Most triptans are available as oral (tablet) formulations. For patients who require a more rapid onset of pain relief, or in whom nausea and vomiting are prominent, other options are available.

Compared to the nonspecific therapies, including analgesics and NSAIDs, triptans provide rapid onset of action (from fifteen minutes to one hour, depending on the formulation), are highly effective in relieving migraine symptoms, and have a favorable side effect profile. Triptans are relatively safe medications compared to the other medications used for acute treatment. In the majority of patients, the intensity of adverse effects is mild and of short duration. People who are at risk for coronary heart disease, diabetes, obesity, severe uncontrolled hypertension, or hypercholesterolemia should be screened prior to administration of triptans.

Even though the triptans have similar basic characteristics, they are different medications from each other. If you do not respond to one triptan, you may respond to another.

Important points to consider:

1. Some of you may not respond to a triptan on the first try. Take it at least two or three times before discarding it.
2. The medication may not work for all migraine attacks.
3. The medication may not provide complete relief of the headache but may decrease the severity of the pain to a more manageable level.
4. For best relief, take the medication at the first symptom of the migraine.
5. Triptans do not prevent recurrence of the headache.

Triptans should not be used for basilar or hemiplegic migraine, if you have heart disease, or if you are taking medications called ergots or monoamine oxidase inhibitors (MAOIs).

Common side effects of triptans:

• chest pressure
• flushing
• dizziness
• drowsiness
• nausea

Recently, the combination of a triptan and a NSAID has been found to be more effective than taking just one of these pain relievers. Treximet is a combination of a triptan, sumatriptan, and naproxen, an NSAID.

Ergotamine
Prior to the introduction of sumatriptan, the most commonly used medication for treating acute migraine attack was ergotamine. In the United States, ergotamine is available under the brand name Cafergot, which is a combination of ergotamine and caffeine. Ergots are available in many different forms: as a pill, sublingual tablet (placed under the tongue), nasal spray, intramuscular or subcutaneous injection, or a rectal pill. The maximum dose is six milligrams in a twenty-four-hour period. As with the triptans, it

should be taken at the first sign of a migraine headache. It is an effective drug, but it should be used with caution.

It has many potential side effects, including nausea, vomiting, diarrhea, and dizziness. In some people, it can cause high blood pressure. It should not be taken on a daily basis, as excessive use can cause a condition known as ergotism, where the blood circulation in the limbs is severely decreased. In addition, medication overuse headaches are commonly seen in patients taking this medication on a regular basis. Daily or very frequent use can also lead to the development of tolerance. Furthermore, it can worsen a condition known as Raynaud's syndrome, where the tips of fingers and toes can turn white, then blue. If you suffer from Raynaud's, you should not use ergots.

In addition, there are many contraindications to the use of ergots. These include heart disease, glaucoma, liver disease, uncontrolled high blood pressure, peripheral vascular diseases, kidney disease, and many others. So, if you are considering using ergots, and you have any of these conditions, discuss your options for pain relief with your doctor before taking this medication.

Dihydroergotamine (DHE)

DHE is a derivative of ergotamine. In the United States, it is available as brand names **DHE-45** and **Migranal**. The DHE-45 is the injectable form of DHE, while Migranal is the nasal spray form. DHE-45 has been used effectively for intractable migraine in its intravenous form. DHE-45 is very effective but has to be given in a hospital setting. It is also used to detoxify patients who are suffering from MOH.

Contraindications to the use of ergotamine or DHE

- heart problems
- severe hypertension
- kidney disease
- liver disease
- recent infection
- pregnancy

Other Medications for Acute Pain

Opioids

In addition to the triptans, many people use narcotic medications, especially when the pain is severe or non-responsive to triptans or NSAIDs. The most common of these medications are the **opioids**. Studies have shown that opioids are effective in pain relief of migraine.

Would you believe that the use of opioids dates back to the seventeenth century at least? Thomas Sydenham, who is known as the Father of English Medicine, or the English Hippocrates, is reported to have said, "Of the remedies it has pleased Almighty God to give to man to relieve his sufferings, none is so universal and efficacious as opium."

Because there can be problems of side effects and the potential for addiction, there are established guidelines for the use of opioids.

Opioids should be used:

1. **Infrequently** in the treatment of moderate-to-severe headaches that are not responsive to standard medications
2. For acute headaches, and only when **non-opioid medication has failed** or is contraindicated. (The principle of stratified care does not apply here, as it can lead to addiction).
3. As **rescue medication** of severe, middle-of-the-night headache
4. When the patient is **pregnant**
5. In patients with no history of drug abuse
6. When use will be limited to one or two treatment days per week

Your doctor should set strict limits and prescribe small amounts to avoid overuse. In cases of menstrual migraine and pregnancy, opioids can be used more frequently. The major concerns of these medications are overuse leading to addiction, drug-induced headache, and withdrawal. Withdrawal symptoms may be minor (restlessness, anxiety, sleep disturbances, tremors, and stomach upset) or major (agitation, delirium, psychosis, abnormally low blood pressure, and seizures). Withdrawal is more likely with short-acting medications. The most commonly used opioid analgesics for migraine are oxycodone by itself or in combination with acetaminophen (brand name Percocet), hydrocodone with acetaminophen (brand names Vicodin, Lortab, Norco, Lorcet), morphine (brand name Kadian, MS Contin), butorphanol (brand name Stadol) and meperidine (brand name Demerol).

Having said that, most headache specialists do not recommend taking opioids for the treatment of headaches. Research has shown that taking opioids more than eight days per month is enough to cause medication-overuse headaches.

Steroids

There is not much scientific data to support the use of steroids in the acute treatment of migraine. The mechanism by which they work is not very clear. It is thought that they decrease inflammation around the blood vessels. They are typically used to break headache cycles. The medication most commonly used is methylprednisolone, also known as the Medrol dose pack, and the intravenous medication dexamethasone (brand name Solumedrol). These are used for atypical migraines.

Antiemetics

In many cases, migraine is accompanied by nausea and/or vomiting. Antiemetics are used not only for their effect on nausea and vomiting, but also for the treatment of headache itself. These medications are generally used in combination with other more specific medications, such as DHE-. In addition, some of the antiemetics (especially the phenothiazines) can cause drowsiness. This sedative effect is useful in relieving the other symptoms associated with migraine. However, there are non-sedating antiemetics, such as trimethobenzamide (brand name Tigan) and metoclopramide (brand name Reglan).

How to choose the right medication

When you are suffering from a headache, all you want is pain relief. An ideal drug is one that provides quick pain relief, prevents recurrence of the headache, has few side effects, if any, and is not costly. So far, the best drugs that have been found to be most effective are the triptans. But if the triptan does not work fully, then adding an antiemetic, such as metoclopramide, can be very helpful. Another option is to add a NSAID, such as naproxen. If you are not able to take a triptan, due to side effects or contraindications, then DHE is a good alternative. The non-specific medications, such as aspirin, acetaminophen, diclofenac, or other NSAIDs can be very effective as well.

Action Exercises

1. Have you taken any medications for acute pain relief? If yes, list all the medications.
2. Have you experienced side effects from the medications? If yes, list all the side effects.
3. Have you ever taken opioids or other narcotics?

CHAPTER 15

Conventional Approach to Headache Treatment: Prophylactic or Preventative Treatment

- Preventative therapy is considered when headaches become too frequent or when acute medications do not work.
- Preventative medications do not work right away; it takes time for the body to acclimate to them.
- When starting preventative medications, the motto is "Start low, go slow."
- Only four medications have been approved by the FDA for migraine prevention as of this writing, but many more are also used off-label.
- Finding the right preventative medication can be complicated; therefore, it is essential to have a partnership with your doctor.

A s a preventive approach, the main objective of prophylactic therapy is to reduce the frequency, intensity, and duration of recurrent attacks. With the advent of triptans and their effectiveness in stopping acute attacks, the use of prophylactic therapy has changed. Treating headaches is not the same thing as preventing them. Treating involves taking a medication to experience immediate relief after a headache starts. The goal of preventative treatment is to reduce the number, intensity, and duration of headaches a person experiences, thus enabling a happier, healthier lifestyle.

It is important to recognize that the goal is not to prevent ALL headaches. It may not be possible to achieve complete freedom from headaches using preventative medications. In fact, if the preventative medication decreases the headache frequency by 50 percent, it is considered a success. Therefore, it is important to have the right expectations; otherwise, you might be sorely disappointed. The secondary goal is to render the acute treatments more effective and to reduce the recurrence.

If your headache characteristics fall into any one of these categories, you are a candidate for preventative therapy:

1. **Frequent headaches**: two or more migraine headaches per month, disabling you for at least three days, which significantly interferes with your daily routine despite adequate use of acute medications
2. **Contraindications to abortive therapy**: you cannot tolerate acute medications, either because you have significant side effects, or the medications are not indicated due to the presence of other medical conditions, or if they are simply not effective in treating the pain
3. **Overuse of abortive therapy**: you are using acute therapy very frequently
4. **Presence of complicated migraine**: you have complicated migraine, such as basilar artery migraine or hemiplegic migraine, where the acute therapies are generally not prescribed

Most of the physicians have reported that only a small percentage of people who might benefit from preventative therapy actually receive it. Some of the most common reasons are:

1. Some people do not want to take a medication every day for something that occurs infrequently.
2. Medications may have side effects.
3. Lack of good response to headache medications in the past, usually due to poor choice of medication, a dose that was too low, inadequate duration of treatment, or poor compliance (people do not take medication as prescribed)
4. Rebound headaches due to overuse of medications, which, instead of helping the patient, are now causing the headache

Lack of education about preventative headache therapy among the general population is also a big factor. Some migraine sufferers do not realize the chronic nature of the disease, focusing only on the episodic nature of their headaches, hoping they will not get their next headache and dreading it because they know they will. If you are utilizing some of the natural treatment modalities to reduce the headache burden, you do not belong to this category, as you are actively addressing the cause of the problem. Some migraine sufferers are concerned about side effects. All migraine preventative drugs can have side effects. However, expert physicians use the medications in ways that can minimize these.

In addition, if you do not understand the basic concept of preventative medications, you may become easily frustrated and give up too soon. Most of the preventative medications belong to one of three categories:

• Antiepileptic (for treating seizures and epilepsy)
• Antidepressant (for treating depression or other mood disorders)

Start Low, Go Slow
1. Start medications at a low dose to allow the body to acclimate to the medication.
2. Increase the dose slowly until a desired target dose is reached.

If one medication does not work, you may need to try a different medication. In fact, several trials may be needed before you find the right preventative medication. The medication is started at a low dose and increased slowly to control the dose-related side effects. Prescribing too much medication from the onset will generally cause too many side effects. The start-low go-slow method might frustrate some people because they are unable to experience an immediate effect from the medication. As the therapeutic level of these medications builds up, they become more effective.

However, you need to keep things in perspective. Even though you need to educate yourself about the possible side effects of the drugs that you may need to take, keep in mind that not everyone gets side effects. In fact, the really serious reactions are very rare. You need to approach this with a positive attitude. If you expect bad things to happen, the chances are they will.

Preventative medications have a great potential for reducing the frequency, intensity, and duration of the headaches. Once the decision has been made to use preventative therapies, a physician can choose from four drugs that have been approved by the US Food and Drug Administration (FDA) for prevention of migraine.

These are:

1. Topiramate (Topamax), an anti-seizure medication
2. Propranolol (Inderal), a blood-pressure-lowering medication
3. Divalproex sodium (Depakote), an anti-seizure medication
4. Timolol (Timolide, Blocadren), a blood-pressure-lowering medication

There is equally strong evidence for the effectiveness and safety among these medications as well as amitriptyline (an antidepressant in frequent use, although not approved by the FDA for migraine prophylaxis).

The American Academy of Neurology (AAN) and the American Headache Society (AHS) have established guidelines for the use of preventative medications based upon available evidence. They have divided the medications into different groups based upon strength of the evidence. The highest recommendations, Level A, are for the four drugs mentioned above (topiramate, propranolol, valproate, and timolol), and a fifth drug, metoprolol, which is another blood-pressure-lowering medication. Amitriptyline is considered a Level B drug.

Anticonvulsants

These medications were originally designed to treat seizures. However, they have been found to be very effective in treating many different conditions, including migraine headaches. Two of these drugs, topiramate and divalproate, have been FDA-approved for this condition, but other medications have also been used with good success. The other aniconvulsant medications sometimes used for migraine prevention include gabapentin (brand name Neurontin), levetiracetam (brand name Keppra), lamotrigine (brand name Lamictal), oxcarbazepine (brand name Trileptal), and pregabalin (brand name Lyrica), although there is no good scientific evidence for their effectiveness.

Topiramate (brand name Topamax)

Topiramate is one of the newer anti-seizure medications. As with other anticonvulsants like divalproex, topiramate has been shown to be effective in the prevention of migraine headaches. The dosages used for migraine prevention are typically less than those required to treat epilepsy. A typical dosage regimen might start with twenty-five milligrams once a day for one week, with the dosage increasing to twenty-five milligrams twice a day. It has been known to cause problems with memory and concentration in some people, as well as tingling in the fingertips. Some patients describe feeling like a zombie with decreased cognitive abilities. In fact, some patients say they feel stupid on the medication. A possibly favorable side effect of topiramate is its effect on weight. It was found that some patients experienced a reduction of approximately 3.8 percent of their body weight.

Some people experience hair loss or thinning hair, and diarrhea. There is also an increased tendency to form kidney stones. Drinking a lot of water, taking the dietary supplement Biotin, and an effective anti-diarrheal medication can help counteract some of these side effects.

Topiramate can also change your sense of taste. Some of you may not be able to drink carbonated beverages anymore, which can be a good thing.

Divalproate

Divalproex sodium, or divalproate (brand name Depakote and Stavzor), is an antiepileptic medication that has been approved by the FDA for migraine prevention. Some migraine patients have an increased tendency to have seizures. There is also an increased incidence of anxiety and depression in patients with migraine headaches. For these people, this medication can be ideal, as it will help these conditions as well. The medication does have side effects, which include nausea, gastrointestinal distress, sedation, tremor, liver toxicity, and some blood disorders. Some people may experience mild weight gain. It is essential to check blood tests before starting treatment and at frequent intervals to monitor any adverse effects of the drug. Liver damage can be serious and fatal, especially during the first six months of treatment. Frequent blood monitoring in the first six months is important.

There is an extended-release preparation of Depakote, which can be taken once daily instead of twice daily for the regular Depakote.

Beta-Blockers:

Propranolol (brand name Inderal) and Timolol

Propranolol belongs to a group of medications called beta-blockers, and is an effective choice of medication for migraine prevention. It is an antihypertensive medication, so it is a good drug if you have high blood pressure or an underlying heart disease and thus may not be able to take triptans or ergots. Common side effects include fatigue, stomach upset, insomnia, hypotension (lowering of blood pressure), decreased heart rate, dizziness, and sexual dysfunction. In people who already have low blood pressure, or who are on many medications for high blood pressure, it should be used with caution. The other medications may need to be adjusted so that the blood pressure does not become too low.

The other beta-blockers have also been shown to have effectiveness in migraine prevention. Timolol and metoprolol (brand name Lopressor or Toprol) have been approved for this indication. Atenolol (brand name Tenormin), has also been used in select patients.

Methysergide (brand name Sansert)

Methysergide is an effective drug for migraine headaches. However, it is not commonly used because it can have toxic side effects. It is a synthetic drug similar to ergotamine, structurally related to the potent hallucinogen LSD. It is used prophylactically to reduce the frequency and intensity of severe migraine headaches. It is similar to sumatriptan in stimulating serotonin receptors. It should be used with caution in patients with heart disease. It interacts with nicotine in promoting the constriction of blood vessels, which can lead to decreased blood flow. Long-term use of methysergide has been associated with production of fibrous tissue of the lining of the kidneys and lungs, and thickening of heart valves. It should not be given to patients who have problems of the heart valves, or who have lung or kidney disease. Common side effects include nausea, vomiting, abdominal pain, drowsiness, leg cramps, numbness, weight gain, and hair loss. It is generally not prescribed for more than four to six months consecutively, with a period of four to six weeks of drug-free interval.

Antidepressants

Antidepressants, especially the tricyclic antidepressants (TCAs), which include amitriptyline (brand name Elavil), nortriptyline (brand name Pamelor), desipramine (brand name Norpramin), doxepin (brand name Sinequan), and imipramine (brand name Tofranil), have all been used for migraine prevention. Their anti-migraine effect is thought to be independent of their antidepressant effect. The TCAs act to block the re-absorption of serotonin. They are not considered the first choice in prevention of migraine, but in some select patients, they can be very useful. Some of these medications can be more sedating than others. They are also associated with many side effects, including constipation, drowsiness, dry mouth, dizziness, sexual problems, urinary retention, and weight gain.

Some of the newer antidepressants, particularly the selective serotonin reuptake inhibitors (SSRIs), such as fluoxetine (brand name Prozac), sertraline (brand name Zoloft), and paroxetine (brand name Paxil) have been used in migraine prevention. However, lack of scientific data limits their use. They have similar side effects to the TCAs. Most other antidepressants have also been used with varying degrees of success.

Calcium channel blockers

Another group of medications that are sometimes used in migraine prevention are calcium-channel blockers, which are frequently prescribed by cardiologists for some heart conditions. These are particularly helpful for hemiplegic migraine and possibly basilar-type migraine. They are also used in migraine with aura. These include verapamil (brand name Calan), nimodipine (brand name Nimotop), and nifedipine (brand names Adalat and Procardia).

Onabotulinumtoxin A (brand name Botox)

Most recently, Botox was approved by the FDA for prevention of chronic migraine headaches. It is an injectable drug, and no pill form is available. It is injected approximately every three months around the head and neck region. It does not seem to work as well for headaches occurring less frequently than fourteen days per month. Botox is made by the company Allergan, and in two studies funded by the company, the drug showed a modest benefit in the prevention of headaches. Keep in mind that Botox must be injected by an experienced physician. Ironically, the most common side effects are neck pain and headache. In some patients, Botox can be very effective when other drugs have not produced significant relief from pain.

How Effective Are the Preventative Medications?

The preventative medications need to be taken for an adequate period of time and with the optimal dose before concluding that they are not effective. Research studies show that 40 to 50 percent of people on preventive medications experience more than a 50 percent decrease in their headaches. The problem with these medications is that they don't always work, and even when they do, they don't always work well. In addition, they may have side effects. There is also some evidence that combining two different preventatives may be more effective, such as a beta-blocker and valproate, or a beta-blocker plus topiramate, but this can increase the incidence of side effects. An important caveat is that you have to try the treatment for an adequate duration and with an adequate dose. A common mistake most people make is to quit taking these medications before they have had a chance to be effective.

Creating a Partnership

Finding the right preventative medication can be complicated. It is vitally important to establish a good working relationship with your health care provider. He or she will spend the time necessary to know you well, including not only your medical history, but also your habits, social involvements, dietary routines, and other factors that can influence the choice of treatment for optimal management of your headache. You need to have a partnership founded on trust, patience, and the knowledge that the physician is committed to finding the right treatment for you whether it is pharmacological, dietary, or an alternative form of treatment.

Action Exercises

1. State in your own words whether you think you are a candidate for preventative therapy, and list your reasons.
2. Does your physician take the time to understand your lifestyle, diet, source of your ailment, and your work environment?
3. Is your physician knowledgeable of alternative medicine and the effects of diet on health?

Section III

NON-PHARMACOLOGIC
TREATMENT OF HEADACHE

CHAPTER 16
Non-Pharmacologic Therapy

- Modern medical treatments are based on evidence-based medicine (EBM), which relies on scientific studies to evaluate the effectiveness of medical treatments.
- Most alternative treatments are not easily tested using EBM.
- Many types of alternative treatments help to restore the body's homeostasis. These include acupuncture, NAET, nutritional approaches, stress and relaxation, lifestyle modification, and homeopathy.

Hundreds of therapies have been used over the centuries for the treatment of headache, ranging from lifestyle changes to aromatherapy to acupuncture to relaxation therapies. In this section, we will explore the non-pharmacologic therapies that have been found to be most effective. An important fact to remember is that these therapies typically address the cause of the headaches, and are not designed merely to provide temporary relief from pain. Due to a general lack of knowledge about alternative medicine, most modern-trained conventional physicians do not routinely prescribe these therapies. However, with the growing realization of the ineffectiveness of conventional strategies, a greater appreciation of alternative approaches is becoming increasingly evident.

The most prevalent approach to choosing a specific treatment is based on evidence-based medicine (EBM). Under EBM, any new treatment, be it medication or a procedure, needs to be studied rigorously in a controlled scientific environment, taking into account any and all biases that may influence the outcome. For any new treatment to be accepted scientifically, and for it to be adopted by the medical community, it is evaluated in terms of type of research studies that have shown its effectiveness in controlling the symptoms of a particular disease, the side-effect profile, and other related aspects. In the evaluation of any new medications for headache, questions are addressed, such as how many patients became headache-free within a certain period, or how many patients experienced a 50 percent reduction in their headaches. Once a drug passes these rigorous trials, it is approved by a regulatory authority such as the FDA for prescribing by physicians.

The irony of this process is that allopathic medications, a term referring broadly to Western or mainstream medicine or other medical procedures, are subject to clinical trials and FDA scrutiny. This means that any other approaches, whether they are supplements, aromatherapy, or acupuncture, are not under the same regulations as pharmaceutical medications. This is both a good and a bad thing. It is good in the sense that there are fewer restrictions on alternative approaches, which means patients do not have to wait for a promising treatment, and bad in the sense that there are fewer restrictions on alternative approaches, which means anyone can market these without any scientific proof of their effectiveness. This makes choosing an alternative therapy more difficult.

The human body carries out its functions primarily in two ways: through chemical and electrical processes. During the last century, Western medicine focused primarily on the chemical nature of disease. This involves determining the ways in which medications can affect the levels of various chemicals in the body, such as hormones and neurotransmitters. In keeping with the Cartesian reductionist view, modern medicine has almost completely ignored the electrical, energetic aspect of medicine. Most modern physicians know very little about the innate healing capacity of the body. Ancient traditional physicians understood the electrical and energetic aspect of medicine, and utilized it in their practice of healing.

Our bodies are miraculous and resilient, and can heal themselves. Alternative approaches primarily support the body's innate corrective programming and natural energy flows to unleash nature's amazing healing power to do its work.

For our purposes, we can divide the various alternative therapies into five major groups:

1. Energy-based medicine, which includes acupuncture and Nambudripad's Allergy Elimination Technique (NAET)
2. Relaxation and stress management
3. Nutritional and herbal approaches
4. Lifestyle modification
5. Other therapies, including homeopathy

In the following pages, we will examine some of these approaches in detail. Before we get into the specific modes of treatment, let us discuss some general principles regarding alternative non-drug therapies.

Principles of Non-Pharmacologic Therapy

There are many causes and types of headaches; however, the majority of them are related in one form or another to a person's lifestyle. Yes, there may be a genetic basis, but environmental factors and personal choices are very closely linked to all forms of primary headaches. As personal lifestyle choices are unique to everyone, treatment needs to be tailored to each individual's situation.

The human body has great healing capacity and a remarkable system for maintaining internal stability, known as homeostasis. In our daily life, we are constantly subjecting our body to extremes of physical, mental, and emotional stress. If we do not provide adequate, proper, and balanced nutrition, physical activity, and stress relief, we can push this remarkable body to its limits, at which point the internal homeostatic mechanisms start to break down, allowing diseases to develop. The aim of these alternative forms of therapy is to bring the body back to its stable internal environment. According to this philosophy, headache is but a symptom of the underlying breakdown of these homeostatic mechanisms.

Modern scientific approach provides a classification for headaches, but in alternative medicine, there is no classification required, as it is believed that all headaches have an underlying cause. Modifying our lifestyle has been shown to be a highly effective treatment strategy regardless of the type of headache we may be suffering from.

In a study conducted at Loma Linda University, Dr. Zuzana Bic, a neurologist and public health specialist, examined the role of lifestyle modification on headache treatment. Dr. Bic showed that lifestyle modification dramatically decreased the frequency, intensity, and duration of headaches in more than 90 percent of patients suffering from migraines. And in many cases, the headaches resolved completely. The study identified three specific areas of lifestyle modification: a balanced nutritional diet low in fat and refined sugar, physical activity, and stress management. The results of the study are given in Appendix 6.

Another caveat of alternative medicine is its basis in the mind-body connection. Ancient medical traditions, including Ayurveda and traditional Chinese medicine (TCM), have recognized the connection of the mind and the body. Recent research at the National Institutes of Health (NIH) has led to important insights into this connection. In simple terms, the mind-body connection describes how our thoughts and emotions affect our body. Each of us is born with a unique constitution, which is expressed in our mental and physical attributes. The cause of our disease lies in this unique constitution.

Disease is the physical manifestation of the breakdown of mental, emotional, and spiritual homeostasis. Whereas conventional medicine describes the differences between diseases, such as tension headache and migraine, alternative medicine assesses the differences between people. Conventional Western medicine determines what *disease* you have. Eastern medicine determines *who you are* in your body, mind, and spirit. In other words, the focus of alternative medicine is the patient and not the disease. This is further exemplified in the instance where two individuals with identical presentation of migraine headache may have two entirely different treatment protocols based on their unique constitution.

Consider your body as a house. This house has a foundation. The strength of the foundation determines the strength of the house. You decide to beautify the house by painting the walls a new color, putting in nice furniture, and hanging beautiful paintings. If that is all that you do, then the house will look nice for a while, but if the foundation is weak, it will soon manifest itself. The windows will not close properly; you may witness leaks in the ceiling, and termites in the floors. Your happiness from the beautification effort will be short lived. When the roof is leaking, the rainy season will be especially uncomfortable. When the windows do not close properly, you will be shivering in the cold weather. And the festering of the termites will soon cause you to fall through holes in the floor. Similarly, if you do not address the foundation of your health, and are only suppressing the symptoms, you may be able to control the headaches for a period, but eventually your overall health will suffer.

The ideal approach is to first fix the foundation and then repair the windows, the floor, and the ceiling before hanging the pictures and arranging new furniture. Similarly in terms of one's health, it is important to assess the cause of the problem so that the solution will have a lasting, long-term effect. The next few pages will address this approach in the management of headache.

CHAPTER 17
Laws of Nature

- A vital energy force animates the physical body. This vital force, known as *prana* in Indian philosophy and Qi in Asian medicine, activates every cell and every tissue within the body.
- The growth and development of every individual depends on the contribution of energy from the three parts of the structure: the physical energy of the body, the dynamic energy of the brain, and the spiritual energy of the spirit.
- Good health is defined as a balanced state of well-being of the body, mind, and soul and not just the absence of disease.
- Disease is a manifestation of an imbalance among vital energies.
- There is a tendency in all living things to respond in a self-curative manner toward illness.

All ancient traditions hold certain wisdom covering many aspects of human life including the cure of diseases. These traditions are based upon natural laws that govern all forms of life in the known universe. From the Ayurvedic traditions of ancient India to Hippocrates, Aristotle, and Paracelsus, to Traditional Chinese Medicine and acupuncture, to the relatively recent advent of homeopathy in the eighteenth century, all can trace their success to recognition of the natural laws that guided the development of their respective doctrines.

However, without understanding the laws that govern nature, our grasp of the ancient wisdom will be superficial.

The first and foremost concept to understand is the concept of life itself. The human body is not just a compilation of mechanical parts that work together in perfect harmony. A vital energy force animates the physical body. This vital force is called *prana* in Indian philosophy, *Qi* (pronounced *chee*) in Asian medicine, *Ki* in Japanese, and *Chai* in Hebrew. In plain English, we call it the soul. This Prana Shakti, or life force, activates every cell and every tissue within the body. This vital force cannot be manufactured or obtained through any artificial means. Without this vital energy, the body becomes inanimate. We are born with this vital force, and it is totally unique to every individual.

The Trinity of Mind, Body, and Spirit

The human organism is a three-part structure of mind, body, and spirit. No organ, tissue, or cell is independent of the activities of the others, and the life of each cell is merged into the life of the whole. The growth and development of every individual depends on the contribution of energy from these three parts of the structure: the physical energy of the body, the dynamic energy of the brain, and the spiritual energy of the spirit. When all three energies work together in harmony, the individual grows and develops normally. Any imbalance between these three vital energy sources results in the manifestation of disease. In other words, *disease is an imbalance of the integrated functioning of the organism and is expressed not only at the physical level, but also at the mental and spiritual levels.*

In practical terms, what that means is that the way we live our life produces either health or disease. As we mentioned in the Introduction, there are three stages of a person's existence: Rajas, Tamas, and Satvik. Which of these stages are you presently at? Is your life controlled by pursuit of worldly pleasures (rajas), or the pursuit of ambition and desires (tamas)? Or, have you reached a state of peace and tranquility (satvik)? When life is lived solely for the purpose of pleasure, ambition, and desire, without regard to the development of the soul, without having a higher purpose, it creates an internal imbalance, which manifests itself as disease.

Every action we take requires the channelization of our internal power. When this power is channeled into activities that promote unhygienic living, both at the physical and mental level, the direction is focused away from activities that promote sound physical and mental health. This wrong focus results in suboptimal energy flow for nourishment and functioning of the internal organs.

Since we know that symptoms are an outward manifestation of imbalance within the body, the suppression of those symptoms does not resolve the underlying problem. This leads to the spread of disease to organs distant from the origin of the disease. Focused reliance on suppressing the symptoms is a major difference between modern and alternative medicine.

Positive Indicators of Health

Good health is defined as *a balanced state of well-being of the body, mind, and soul, and not just the absence of disease.* In this state of good health, all the organ systems work in harmony with one another. When there is balance, there is *ease.* When the organs are out of balance, there is initially *unease*, which can develop into *disease.* Headache is a manifestation of either *unease* or *disease*, and as such, is an excellent initial indicator of a disruption in the natural flow of energy.

When a person becomes diseased, the expression of this vital energy is changed. There is a sense of discomfort. Physical signs and symptoms appear. This process can fester on a low-grade level until some disturbance interacts with the disturbed vital energy, leading to a sudden burst of symptoms that we see as manifestations of acute disease.

You can assess your level of health by examining the following positive indicators:

Physical

1. Evenness in the distribution of heat (body temperature)
2. A unique sense of lightness
3. A general feeling of comfort at all times
4. A keen hunger with good digestion
5. Deep sleep every night (number of hours depends on the individual) and waking in the morning with a feeling of freshness and energy.
6. All the body parts function smoothly and efficiently.
7. All the eliminatory functions of the bowel, bladder, skin, and lungs are carried out easily and with minimal discomfort. This maintains internal cleanliness.

Mental

1. Optimistic outlook on life
2. Having a good sense of humor
3. Able to fully express your unique creativity
4. Following your life purpose
5. Clarity of mind, where the mind is cool, calm, and composed
6. Right attitude toward work—all the worldly activities are performed with a good attitude

Emotional

1. Doing what you love
2. Experiencing a childlike expression of joy
3. Having the capacity to express, experience, and accept feelings of joy and pain
4. Experiencing a sense of accomplishment on a regular basis
5. Not hindered by fear

Spiritual

1. Having a relationship with a higher power
2. Following your intuition

3. Having a sense of gratitude
4. Having a sense of inner peace

The vital force always wants to get back into a state of balance or homeostasis. It is a fundamental law that *all living things tend to respond in a self-curative manner toward illness.* As the vital force attempts to restore normalcy and recover from the diseased state, the symptoms slowly start to improve.

It is interesting and important to note that symptoms resolve in the reverse order of their appearance.

The vital force permeates all forms and degrees of life and is the fundamental of all the conditions of the universe. The same laws apply to humans, with one big difference: the right of choice. Humans exercise this right to the fullest and often choose to go against natural laws. This breach results in imbalance of the energies. The *holistic* approach recognizes this imbalance and tries to help the self-healing powers to fulfill their duty.

In natural medicine, diseases are divided into two categories: acute and chronic.

- **Acute diseases** are defined as processes where the vital force is so overcome as to be unable to restore balance. They can range from mild to severe. If the acute disease is merely suppressed with medication without addressing the underlying cause, then the acute disease can become chronic.
- **Chronic diseases** are conditions where the patient is not able to restore balance to the vital power over an extended period. In these states, the vital force is unable to rectify the condition without external assistance.

Action Exercises

1. Do you feel increased anxiety or stress before experiencing your headache?
2. Does your headache occur before a particularly stressful event?
3. Have you observed a change in habit or diet recently, which might be a cause for imbalance of your vital energies?

CHAPTER 18

Effect of Mind on Health

- There is an intimate relationship between the mind and the body; the mind determines either health or disease.
- The outward physical reality is a reflection of your inner reality, your mind, and your spirit.
- You can control your headaches and maintain good health by changing your thoughts.
- Disease occurs because of your inability to recognize the true essence of who you are.

U ltimately, the mind is the pivotal point of health or disease. This fact may be hard to accept by some, but there is increasing evidence that what has been recognized for centuries by ancient societies is being borne out in scientific studies. The emerging new medical field of *psychoneuroimmunology* is based on the premise that there is an intimate relationship between the mind and body, specifically the effect of emotions on the development of health and illness. This seemingly complicated word describes how the psyche (mind) affects the nervous system (the brain), and how they both affect the immune system. When the mind is discontent and is constantly craving instant gratification, or is under the influence of excessive negative emotions, such as anger, guilt, hate, chronic unhappiness, fear, and shame, this can turn inward and cause an imbalance in the energy flow. Initially, the disease is in a *latent* form, where there are little or no overt symptoms. Headache is a common initial symptom of this latent disease, and as such, can act as a warning of an underlying onset of energy imbalance. Emotional stress leads to a complicated cascade of physical and biochemical responses, all of which affect the function of the major organs and the integrity of the immune system.

Sigmund Freud developed the concepts of the unconscious mind and believed that emotions frequently become repressed in the unconscious. It is now recognized that early childhood emotional trauma can result in many diseases later on in life. In our experience, this is an important aspect of people suffering from all types of headaches. Emotional stress causes a slow deterioration in the functioning of the brain. When emotions are repressed, the immune system becomes affected to such a degree that it is not able to protect the body against illness. In many cases, chronic pain is rooted in the unconscious mind. Physical symptoms are usually a reaction to these unconscious feelings.

There are four possible causes of this emotional trauma:

1. Early childhood adverse experiences, such as physical, emotional, verbal and/or sexual abuse, neglect, and loss of one or both parents from divorce or death
2. Self-imposed pressure, such as in perfectionists who are never able to meet their own standards
3. Abnormally increased reaction to the pressures of daily life
4. Even when there has been no neglect or abuse, emotional trauma can occur when something positive is withheld. The absence of positive stimuli, whether real or perceived, is an important cause of emotional trauma.

As the negative emotion manifests as stress and builds over time without any form of significant release, it accumulates and becomes stronger. It eventually reaches a critical threshold, where it starts producing physical symptoms. The internal environment becomes disordered, and the individual becomes vulnerable to various diseases. Headache is an early manifestation of a disturbed internal environment. Of particular importance is the repression of anger, which greatly increases physiological stress.

According to most spiritual traditions, the outward physical reality is, in fact, a reflection of your inner reality, your mind. You perceive reality from your own perspective. A singular event can be interpreted in different ways depending on the perspective of the observers. For example, if we were to pour a jug of water on two people, we might get a completely different response from each individual. One person might get upset because he or she dislikes getting wet, while the other person might have a laugh and feel that the water is refreshing. In effect, the cause, in this instance, the pouring of water, has two different effects depending on the perspective of the person. Reality, therefore, is subjective, and is dependent on the way your mind perceives it. A happy person views the world as a happy place, and an unhappy person sees the world as full of suffering.

Swami Vivekananda, a well-known yogi, states:

"This world has no existence. What is meant by that? It means that it has no absolute existence. It exists only in relation to my mind, to your mind, and to the mind of else. We see this world with the five senses, but if we had another Sense, we would see in it something more. If we have yet another Sense, it would appear as something still different. It has, therefore, no real existence."

The state of mind depends on one's beliefs and convictions. The outer reality is a product of your thought waves. An unfocused mind generally tends to attract negative thoughts more often, and as a result, the mind's reality tends to be pessimistic and unhealthy. In this state, discontent, sickness, and disease are different forms of the same reality. The good news is that one can convert this pessimistic unhealthy state of mind into eternal optimism, vibrant health, and happiness just by changing one's thoughts and inner reality, where pain and suffering do not exist.

This concept has far-reaching consequences for how you live life. Many motivational thinkers and teachers have recognized that the power of the mind can be utilized in programming your brain to produce success and wealth. In other words, your mind creates your reality. Likewise, your mind attracts health or disease. If your reality has created headaches, then the only way to get rid of the headaches completely is by changing your inner reality, by learning the laws of nature and following them. While it is beyond the scope of this book to engage in a lengthy discourse on the topic, living according to a purposeful lifestyle such as described by Bhai Gurdas, a Sikh poet from India, may help you to achieve eternal health and happiness. Interested readers are encouraged to explore such concepts further by learning about great spiritual teachers and thinkers from the Eastern traditions.

Bhai Gurdas explains this concept of healthy living in a verse, which I have translated here:

Wake up in the early hours of the morning, bathe yourself, and meditate.
Speak kind words, have humility, and give of yourself for the wellbeing of others.
Sleep, eat, and speak only in moderation; this is the way of the godly person.
Earn an honest day's labor; be big of heart but not big of ego.
Keep the company of godly people, and live by these principles day and night.
Meditate daily, and be happy and content with what life has to offer.
Remain detached amid hopes and desires.

Why Does One Get Diseases?

Where there is health, there is no disease, and where there is disease, there is no health. The biggest cause of pain and suffering in the world is disease. Disease does not discriminate: it affects the rich and the poor, the learned and the illiterate. People spend a great portion of their hard-earned money on medicines and visits to hospitals, doctors, and clinics. Only a very lucky few have escaped the grip of disease. This raises the question: Is there no cure for this problem?

Why are we destined to suffer from diseases, often with no recourse? Why does disease occur in the first place?

According to most spiritual philosophies, disease occurs because of our inability to recognize the true essence of who we are. People who have recognized their true essence find the cure for the diseases within themselves. They recognize the unseen force that exists within them (and everyone), and are able to access it to rid themselves of disease. The answer lies in recognizing this innate power. When you can access this unseen power, you can utilize it to cure yourself of suffering. **Guru Nanak**, founder of the Sikh faith, addressed this issue in a verse, which is translated below:

> *When you are plagued by great and excessive anxiety, and diseases of the body*
> *When you are wrapped up in the attachments of household and family, sometimes feeling joy, and other times sorrow*
> *When you are wandering around in all four directions, and you cannot sit or sleep even for a moment*
> *If you come to remember the Supreme Lord God, then your body and mind shall be cooled and soothed.*

The word *healing* means *whole*. It can be said that to be truly healed is to become whole. When internal harmony is amiss or disturbed, one is in a state of less than whole. Real healing takes place when the internal harmony is reestablished.

Finding Your True Identity

There is a great misconception in the world as to what constitutes a person. Almost everyone perceives him or herself to be the physical manifestation of a person, and as such, one is a living, breathing, doing, and thinking body that can feel and experience pain and suffering or pleasure and happiness. When you are sick, you will generally state, "I am not well," or "I am suffering," or "I have a headache." This is because we feel that we are only our body.

Consider the following example. When you undergo a surgical operation, an anesthesiologist gives you an anesthetic agent to make you unconscious. In that state of unconsciousness, a surgeon can cut any part of your body, and you will not feel any pain whatsoever. If the body were a living, breathing entity, then you would experience all pain regardless of anesthesia. The body, in and of itself, is not what is alive. Along this line of reasoning, as with all such lifeless substances, the body does not get sick. If that is the case, then who becomes sick? Who suffers pain? Who gets heart disease or cancer? To answer that question, we have to understand the concept of the soul, also referred to as the spirit, which resides in each of us, and the mind.

Every spiritual philosophy has recognized this entity as the essence of one's being. Most consider it immortal; some even believe that it does not suffer and does not get sick. If you really think about it, you will realize that the entity that generally gets sick and experiences pain and suffering is your mind.

What is the mind? Your mind is a collection of your thoughts and views of life. If your thoughts are pure, your mind is pure. If that is true, then the mind can recover from illness. Since the mind is a repository of thoughts, whatever the mind thinks, it experiences. If the mind has happy thoughts, the mind becomes happy; if the thoughts are sad, depressing, and fearful, the mind suffers. All aspects of the external world are experienced as thoughts by the mind. Whenever the mind experiences a thought, it creates a mental picture. If you think of a snake, you will create a mental picture of a snake, which then creates a feeling of fear.

Where the mind has the power to create its own thoughts and create mental pictures from these thoughts, it also has the power to prevent the thoughts from occurring. External events can influence the mind only if it lets them. If the mind so chooses, it can shut off thoughts or replace them with other thoughts so that external events have little or no influence on it. The physical body is under the control of these thoughts. The stress response is an example. When you are confronted with a life-threatening situation such as suddenly facing a tiger while you are jogging through the woods, the mind first creates the fear inside, and then this fear creates physical responses. The body in and of itself does not feel fear, but when the mind experiences fear, it creates the corresponding physical responses. When the fear disappears, the body returns to a normal state of calm. Disease attacks the mind first, creating thoughts of fear and anxiety, which in turn create mental pictures from these thoughts, which subsequently affect the body. The weaker the mind, the more susceptible the body is to disease, as the mind in that state cannot create images of well-being, health, and fearlessness.

A strong mind will not allow images of disease and sickness to enter into consciousness. This may be difficult to accept since the mind is not what is suffering from cancer or heart disease, or the other diseases that affect the physical body. However, the mind is the cause; what happens to the body is the effect.

The mind has only one method of preventing these negative thought images and that is by creating positive thought images. The most prevalent thoughts will dictate the effect on the mind and thus the person's reality.

In the ensuing chapters, we will learn how you can change your life by changing your thoughts.

CHAPTER 19
Chinese Medicine and Headaches

- Traditional Chinese Medicine is based on the theory of yin and yang, which sees the body as a whole system, the parts of which are dependent on each other just like a well-balanced ecosystem.
- Acupuncture is the stimulation of specific points in or on the surface of the skin that have the ability to move and direct the flow of qi (life force).
- An acupuncturist extrapolates a pattern based on your symptoms, which points to the origin of the problem. Different patients with the same type of headache may have different patterns and therefore require different treatments.

Brief History of Traditional Chinese Medicine (TCM)

Traditional Chinese Medicine (TCM) dates back four thousand years. The earliest written history of TCM is recorded in a book called *Huangdi Neijing* (221 BC–206 BC). It is a conversation between the emperor and his physician on their theories of illness and treatments. Many of the same ideas are still used today. Unlike modern medicine, which is based on observed facts and physiological theories, TCM is rooted in Confucian and Daoist philosophies. Confucianism believes in feudal and totalitarian systems, which in terms of medicine links internal diseases with external means. Daoism believes in maintaining harmony between man and the world, between this world and beyond, a perfect harmony between opposing forces in nature. This brings us to the theory of yin and yang.

Yin and Yang

Yin and yang is a concept of opposites (hot/cold; night/day; top/bottom; movement/stillness). According to this theory, everything is interdependent and interchanging. It is the fundamental fluctuating balance of nature. TCM sees the body not as parts that can be replaced or removed, but as a whole system whose parts are dependent and interdependent on each other just like a well-balanced ecosystem. For this simple reason, TCM is considered a great preventative medicine.

The concept of hormones, enzymes, allergens, bacteria, viruses and other pathogens does not exist in TCM. What can be seen and felt is Qi. As mentioned earlier, Qi is the energy that flows through channels known as meridians that connect all of our major organs. Qi is the energy that makes the body function properly. When it flows freely, we are healthy. There is a Chinese saying: "Where there is free flow there is no pain; where there is no free flow, there is pain." The meridians in our body act as a freeway system. They transport qi, blood, and other substances to where they are supposed to go. When the flow of qi is impeded, obstructed, or depleted through lack of exercise, poor diet, excess emotions, or trauma, then illness develops. Through TCM, the free flow of qi can again be restored.

TCM incorporates acupuncture, Chinese herbs, and nutrition. Acupuncture is the stimulation of specific points in or on the surface of the skin that have the ability to move and direct the flow of qi. In simple terms, these specific points alter various biochemical and physiological conditions in order to achieve the desired effect. Acupuncture points are areas of designated electrical sensitivity. Inserting needles at these points stimulates various sensory receptors, which, in turn, stimulate nerves that transmit impulses to the *hypothalamic-pituitary system* at the base of the brain.

The hypothalamus-pituitary glands are responsible for releasing neurotransmitters and endorphins, the body's natural pain-killing hormones. It is estimated that endorphins are two hundred times more potent than morphine. Endorphins also play a big role in the functioning of the hormonal system. This is why acupuncture works well for conditions such as headache, back pain, arthritis, premenstrual syndrome, and infertility. The substances released from the correct application of acupuncture not only relax the whole body, but also regulate hormones and neurotransmitters such as serotonin in the brain, thereby positively affecting human and animal disposition. This is why depression is often treated with acupuncture. It also illustrates how the electrical flow within the body affects the body's chemical balance.

Some of the physiological effects of acupuncture that have been observed include increased circulation, decreased inflammation, relief from pain, relief of muscle spasms, and increased T-cell count (which is a reflection of the integrity of the immune system).

There are over three hundred known acupuncture points throughout the body, and they all have their own functions. For example, *large intestine 4*— the highest acupuncture point on the web of the thumb and forefinger of the hand—is commonly known to help with treatment of headaches as it is the command point for the face, mouth, jaw, and nose. Often acupuncture points are combined in a treatment, as they create specific functions associated with each point combination. For example, when *large intestine 4* is combined with a point called *liver 3*, labor is facilitated during childbirth. The acupuncturist is like a traffic controller who directs energy through the meridians for the specific condition that needs to be addressed and thereby balances the energy in a specific area.

Unlike conventional medicine, TCM does not take a patient's symptoms and put a disease or illness label on it. An experienced acupuncturist first takes your history, which includes your current symptoms, physical state, and lifestyle, and extrapolates a pattern. This pattern usually points to the origin (root) of the problem and the condition of the body at present (branch).

Each treatment addresses the root (cause) and branch (presenting symptoms) of the problem. Pattern diagnosis allows you to receive an individualized treatment for your problems. An example of pattern diagnosis can be seen with three patients who have frontal headaches. One person has missed lunch because he worked through his lunch break. Another person has a new baby and only had two hours of sleep the previous night. The third person has demanding work and personal issues that he is trying to sort out. Would it make sense to give painkillers for the headaches? Yes, if you only want to treat the branch of the problem. To treat the source of the problem, the first patient needs to eat something right away, the second needs a good night's sleep, and the third needs to learn stress coping mechanisms. Alternatively, if three people experience different symptoms but they all present the same pattern, then they will receive the same treatment. This is exactly how pattern diagnosis and treatment work.

Chinese Herbal Medicine

Chinese herbal medicine has been around for as long as acupuncture. It is used alone or in conjunction with acupuncture to help with specific conditions. In this context, the term herbal does not refer to supplements or cooking herbs such as oregano or parsley. Chinese medicinal herbs are extracted from plants, minerals, and animals. Herbs are usually not taken alone but as part of a formula, a compilation of single herbs for a specific diagnosis. It is more beneficial to take a formula rather than a single herb because herbs work synergistically, thus minimizing adverse effects. The practitioner will prescribe the type that best suits your pattern. Herbs are especially useful in chronic illnesses such as allergies, headaches, and arthritis.

Herbs come in many forms: raw (the leaves, twigs, and flowers are visible), powder, tinctures (alcohol based), pills, tablets, and capsules. Many people take over-the-counter herbs such as ginseng and gingko biloba. This is not necessarily beneficial for the individual especially if his or her disease pattern does not call for that herb. Chinese herbs are different from other herbs because different parts of a plant provide different medicinal properties; therefore, taking these herbs when they are not indicated may not be beneficial and in fact may be harmful.

Let us take, for instance, the mulberry tree (Latin: *Mori albae*). Each part of the tree can be used for very different conditions. The leaves (Latin: *Folium mori albae*; Chinese: *Sang Ye*) are used in formulas that address lung conditions due to colds and flus where there is thick yellow sputum. They can be used for red, sore, dry, or painful eyes and in mild cases of vomiting blood. The mulberry twigs (Latin: *Ramulus mori albae*; Chinese: *Sang Zhi*) are used for upper extremity joint problems and edema (swelling). The bark of the tree (Latin: *Cortex mori albae readicis*; Chinese: *Sang Bai Pi*) can be used to stop cough and wheezing, swelling of the extremities, fever, thirst, and hypertension. Lastly, the mulberry fruit (Latin: *Fructus mori albae*; Chinese: *Sang Shen*) is used for dizziness, tinnitus, premature graying of hair, and constipation due to blood and yin deficiency patterns.

If you just purchase mulberry extracts from the store without knowing whether whole or part of the plant was used to produce them, and your pattern does not fit even though your symptoms do, you can cause further imbalance to your system and do more harm than good. Herbal medicine does not replace hormones or chemicals in your body, which means that many patients may not feel a strong or immediate affect after taking the herbs. Because of this, they tend to think, *Oh, this can't really hurt me.* They continue taking it not really feeling the negative effects until those become very pronounced. The condition then is much more difficult to reverse.

Many herbs and herbal formulas target head pain even under the same pattern. This is when in-depth knowledge of herbs comes in handy—to be able to direct the herbs to the desired area for treatment. Chinese herbs are not always made from exotic plants; they can be derived from everyday food items you are already familiar with such as ginger, cinnamon, and green onions.

For example, here are some single herbs that can target specific areas of the head:

- **Qiang Huo** (*rhizoma et radix notopterygii*) for occipital headaches
- **Gao Ben** (*rhizoma et radix ligustici*) for vertex headaches
- **Bai Zhi** (*radix angelicae dahuricae*) for supraorbital/frontal headaches

Chinese Medicine—Preventative Therapies

TCM can be used as a good preventative medicine. Are you proactive or reactive when it comes to your health? Most people are reactive; they do not seek help until they are in extreme pain, or when a family member is fed up with their condition and forces them to seek professional advice. You may be getting a complete checkup every year. However, it is ironic that most people treat their cars a lot better than they treat their bodies. Do you only take your car in for its 30,000-, 60,000-, and 90,000-mile tune-ups? Or do you take it in for oil changes and tire rotations every three to five thousand miles? If so, you probably do this to prevent an unexpected breakdown. Your body is a machine that operates like a car. If your energy is off balance, but it is not bad enough for you to notice anything extreme, you tend to think that you are okay and healthy. Then one day you wake up and something is not right anymore. When it gets to this point, treatment will not be as easy as it would have been if you had sought help earlier.

TCM treatments have a cumulative effect over time. The treatment is like pages in a book; alone they seem small and not very significant, but when you put them together, they can make an impressive novel. When your body is a little off balance, it is easy and quick for your health practitioner to bring it back to harmony, but when there is a huge imbalance, it will take some time and great effort to reverse the effects. This proactive mentality is not the norm, so you must incorporate it into your life and act on it. The best thing to do is to seek out a licensed practitioner in your area who has been through a comprehensive four-year program. Be sure to ask lots of questions and be involved in your health. This is the only way you will see results and maintain a healthy life.

Action Exercises

1. Are you proactive or reactive when it comes to your health? Do you take steps to prevent disease, or do you only think about your health when your body starts to break down?

2. Have you experienced acupuncture? Did it provide any relief, even if only temporary?

3. Are you taking any herbs? If so, do you know what they contain? If you don't, ask your health practitioner about them.

CHAPTER 20
Allergy Elimination

- NAET is a non-invasive, drug free, natural solution to eliminate allergies.
- An allergy is a condition of unusual sensitivity of an individual to one or more substances.
- Contact with an allergen produces a blockage in the energy flow through the various energy pathways, or meridians, which presents as an allergy. Headache can also be an allergic reaction.
- NAET utilizes the Neuromuscular Sensitivity Testing (NST), which is a natural, drugless, painless, non-invasive method that can be used safely to discover and treat hidden allergies.
- Almost any substance can be tested using NST.
- The NAET treatment involves stimulating certain key acupuncture spinal points while the patient holds the allergen in his or her hand.

Now that we have an idea about Traditional Chinese Medicine and acupuncture, let us take it a step further. Chinese energy meridian theory has given birth to a recent revolutionary treatment known as Nambudripad's Allergy Elimination Technique (NAET). As the name suggests, this technique was developed by Dr. Devi Nambudripad, MD, DC, LAc, PhD. According to Dr. Devi, NAET is *a non-invasive, drug free, natural solution to eliminate allergies of all types and intensities using a blend of selective testing and energy balancing procedures taken from those practiced in acupuncture/acupressure, allopathy, chiropractic, nutritional, and kinesiological disciplines of medicine.*

Before we get to the details of NAET, it is important to understand the concept of allergy.

According to NAET, an allergy is *a condition of unusual sensitivity of an individual to one or more substances* (whether inhaled, swallowed, or coming in contact with the skin) that may be harmless or even beneficial to the majority of other individuals. In sensitive individuals, contact with these substances (known as allergens) can produce a variety of symptoms including headache. According to Oriental medicine, contact with an allergen produces a blockage in the energy flow through the various meridians (energy pathways). Under normal circumstances, there is a perfect balance of the two types of energies, the yin and the yang. Any imbalance in this yin-yang state causes an energy difference, which manifests itself as an allergy. Most people think of an allergy as a runny nose or sneezing or hives or difficulty breathing, but as you might have guessed by now, headache can also be an allergic reaction. In other words, an allergy is any abnormal response to an allergen.

What Is an Allergy?

An allergy is *a condition of unusual sensitivity of an individual to one or more substances* that may be harmless or even beneficial to the majority of other individuals.

Some people might confuse allergy with hypersensitivity, but there is a difference between the two in the degree of response.

True allergy is the activation of the immune system, consisting of substances in the body known as immunoglobulin type E (IgE) antibodies. This is what is commonly accepted as allergy in Western medicine.

Hypersensitivities, or simply sensitivities, and intolerances are non-IgE-mediated reactions, which produce similar symptoms.

For our purposes, we will use the more general definition of allergy.

In pathophysiological terms, migraine headache is characterized by an oversensitivity of the nervous system to both internal and external triggers. In this context, we can think of triggers as allergens, since these triggers elicit a response from the brain that begins the cascade that leads to the headache. According to NAET, there are different types of allergens or triggers:

1. **Inhalants**: substances that can be inhaled such as dust, pollens, perfumes, paint fumes, and smoke
2. **Contactants**: substances that people can touch or come in contact with, such as fabrics, chemicals, and cosmetics
3. **Infectants**: infectious agents such as bacteria and viruses
4. **Ingestants**: substances that can be ingested or swallowed, such as food, drinks, medications, and drugs
5. **Injectants**: substances that can be injected, such as insect bites, medications, and immunizations
6. **Physical agents**: environmental factors, such as heat, cold, humidity, dampness, wind, dryness, sunlight, and sound
7. **Molds** and **fungi**
8. **Genetic factors**: inherited illnesses or sensitivities
9. **Emotional factors**: usually painful memories of past incidents

Most of these substances can act as triggers for your headache. In some cases, the correlation between the symptom and the allergen is obvious. However, some of you may have never noticed any correlation. Even in less obvious cases, treating for the most common allergens has proven beneficial in treating headaches.

The fact that you may not have noticed any allergens in your particular case, or that we may not be able to identify an allergen by our standard repertoire of diagnostic tests, does not mean that you do not have allergies. The fact is that there are many undiagnosed allergies hiding beneath the majority of unresolved health problems.

Why We Develop Allergies

To understand how and why we develop allergies, we need to digress a bit and understand what good health is and how we achieve it. We all know that one of the secrets to good health is proper nutrition. Proper nutrition in this context is food that can be assimilated by the body easily without causing any discomfort or negative reactions. According to this definition, even foods that we know are good for us, such as fruits and vegetables, may not provide proper nutrition if the body reacts in a negative way when we eat them.

As we saw in the previous chapter, everything we do and eat produces a specific energy in our body. When a person comes into contact with a substance that is not compatible with his or her energy, an energy disturbance takes place. When two adverse energies are present, they repel each other. For example, if someone has an allergy to peanuts, even smelling them can lead to adverse symptoms.

Constant exposure to energies to which a person is averse can ultimately lead to weakening of the person's energy. Energy imbalances are also produced in our relationships. Whenever there is tension or disharmony between two people, it creates an energy imbalance. If a person is constantly surrounded by adverse substances, people, or circumstances, that person's energy becomes weaker with time, leading to further energy imbalance, and ultimately resulting in blockage in the energy flow.

The continuous blockage of the energy pathways leads to altered body function and disease. The weakest parts of the body become affected by the energy blockages first. If the stomach happens to be the weakest part of the body, the person usually gets either abdominal symptoms or headaches. According to

TCM and other natural disciplines, this is one of the major reasons migraines are linked to so many food allergies.

Every one of us has energy imbalances. *Diseases occur when genetic predispositions are combined with energy imbalances.* The more imbalanced the energy, the more likely a person is to have symptoms.

The most common allergens are:

1. foods
2. chemicals (both internal and external)
3. pollen and other environmental substances (both natural, such as trees, grass, and flowers, and man-made, such as chemicals, pesticides, and paint fumes)
4. animals
5. emotions
6. other people

As you can well surmise, a majority of the diseases that affect human beings can be ascribed to these allergies; the symptoms in a particular patient depend on the person's weakest areas of the body. Therefore, allergies to different substances can lead to the same problem in different people, or, conversely, allergy to the same substance can cause different symptoms in different people. Some people react to a combination of these, and some are sensitive to almost anything.

Determining What We Are Allergic To

According to conventional Western medicine, there are several methods for testing allergies. These include the intra-dermal test, the patch test, the scratch test, and various blood tests such as the RAST test and the ELISA test. These can identify dozens of common allergens. The accuracy of these tests is variable.

To some extent, we may be able to recognize which substances are potential allergens, as in the case of migraine triggers. However, since the symptoms developed in an individual may be unique to that individual, we need a more reliable and accurate method of assessing whether a substance is a potential allergen. NAET utilizes one such tool that can be used reliably to identify allergens.

In NAET, the most commonly utilized test is the Neuromuscular Sensitivity Test (NST), which is based on kinesiology. NST is a natural, drugless, painless, non-invasive method that can be used safely in humans, including newborn infants and the elderly, to discover and treat hidden allergies that might cause disease in the future. When an allergen causes an energy blockage in the meridians, the brain sends messages that are manifested as weakness in the muscles, aches/pains, insomnia, depression, headaches, and a variety of other diseases. NST can be reliably used to identify allergens by utilizing the effect of energy blockage on the musculoskeletal system. NAET can then reduce or eliminate allergies to the items identified by this method.

There are many different versions of NST. However, we will discuss the basic principles behind it to help you understand how it works. It is a simple procedure that everyone can and should learn in order to identify substances that are allergens for them. The basis for NST is that when you are exposed to a substance that you are allergic to, one of the changes that take place in your body is that your muscles become weak. The reason behind this muscle weakening effect is the incompatibility of the electromagnetic energy of the substance and the person, resulting in repulsion.

Standard Neuromuscular Sensitivity Test
The following is adapted from the book *Say Goodbye to Illness*. Two people are required for this procedure:

- The patient lies on a table with one arm raised 45 to 90 degrees with the palm facing outward and the thumb facing the big toe.
- The tester stands on the patient's right side.
- The tester tries to push the raised arm of the patient down toward the patient's toe while the patient actively resists the pressure. If the muscle remains strong, the patient is well balanced at the time of testing. If the arm becomes weak without the patient being exposed to the potential allergen, then either the tester is not performing the

test properly or the patient is not well balanced.

- If the muscle remains strong, the tester places the potential allergen in the patient's resting hand.

- The tester again tries to push the raised hand downward. If the potential allergen has electrical charges that are incompatible with the patient's energy, there is an imbalance of the energy, and the muscle becomes weak. This indicates that the patient is allergic to that object. Conversely, if the arm remains strong, the patient is not allergic to that object.

Fortunately, in most people, the immune system is strong and the energy imbalances are mild. Constant bombardment over time, though, can lead to weakening of our body's homeostasis. This is one explanation of why people develop chronic diseases as they grow older.

You may be wondering how the acupuncturist can check for your specific allergens if your body is constantly bombarded with several potential allergens.

The Basic Items

There is a systematic method of identifying the allergens causing your headaches. As a general rule, all of us are exposed to certain common substances on a daily basis. We all eat food. But what we eat differs from individual to individual. Some people are vegetarians, and others are not. Some people have very healthy diets, while others munch on junk food. However, we can break down the food into its various constituents, which include proteins, carbohydrates, minerals, fats, grains, sugars, iron, salt, spices, and so on.

Almost any substance can be tested using NST. However, for practical purposes, Dr. Devi has devised a list of the most common substances that have been implicated in causing allergies. Almost everyone is exposed to these foods and substances on a regular basis.

The Basic List
1. Eggs
2. Calcium

3. Vitamin C
4. Vitamin B complex
5. Sugar
6. Iron
7. Vitamin A
8. Minerals
9. Salt
10. Grains
11. Yeast
12. Acid
13. Base
14. Artificial sweeteners
15. Caffeine / Coffee / Chocolate
16. Nuts
17. Spices
18. Fish and shellfish
19. Animal and vegetable fats
20. Fluoride

To Treat or Not to Treat

Once you have determined potential allergens, the next step is to treat. After all, NAET is not limited to just identifying the potential offending substances. This is what sets NAET apart from other treatment modalities.

Once the NST identifies allergy to a specific substance, this substance is treated by the method developed by Dr. Devi. The NAET Treatment involves stimulating certain key acupuncture spinal points while holding the allergen in your hand. The treatment is non-invasive and involves tapping at specific nerve roots along the spine, followed by stimulating certain key acupuncture points on the limbs, called gate points. The stimulation of these key points is thought to release certain neurochemicals that act as antidotes to the allergen, thus neutralizing the threat. When the body is exposed to the same allergen again, the body remembers it and no longer produces a reaction to it. Patients are told to avoid the treated substance for a certain period after the treatment and then to slowly incorporate it into their daily lives.

Allergic reactions are **not** due to any inherent properties of the substances themselves but are the result of the wrong messages transmitted by the central nervous system. When the signals are reprogrammed, the substance ceases to cause the reactions it caused prior to treatment.

If you are sensitive to multiple allergens, they are treated one at a time. For most substances, the allergic reaction can be eliminated with one treatment cycle. A majority of patients undergoing NAET treatment will notice at least some improvement in their symptoms after completing the treatment of fifteen to twenty substances in the Basic List. Some patients may be highly allergic to one or more items, and for these substances, they may need more than one treatment. For instance, someone allergic to sugar may require two to five treatments for sugar alone. After the treatment, NST is performed again to check if there is recurrence of the symptoms.

Potential Reactions after NAET Treatment

Some people may respond in a positive way immediately after their treatment while others may experience tiredness or fatigue. Others may not experience any improvement initially, but as they go through the basic treatments, they will notice increasing episodes of feeling good. Some people experience a significant craving for the substance being avoided. For instance, if you have an allergy to sugar, you may experience a great craving for sweets during the avoidance period.

NAET treatments have a cumulative effect over time. As more and more of the allergens are eliminated, the immune system becomes stronger and stronger, allowing the body's own healing energies to bring the body back to a state of homeostasis.

Many people's intractable headaches have resolved completely once their triggering allergens were identified using NST and treated with the NAET protocol. In many cases, patients have been able to completely eliminate the use of medications and have achieved true headache freedom.

Action Exercises

1. Have you noticed any particular foods or substances that trigger your headaches?

2. With the help of a friend, perform NST using different substances that you suspect cause your headaches.

CHAPTER 21
Stress: Negative Mind Over Matter

- The fight-or-flight response is our body's primitive, automatic, inborn response that prepares the body to fight or flee from real or perceived attack, harm, or threat to our survival.
- As stress builds up, our body produces the hormones epinephrine and norepinephrine, which give our bodies a surge of adrenaline.
- The body also produces cortisol, which limits the adrenaline response.
- Chronic stress keeps the cortisol level elevated. Treatment should be aimed at identifying the cause of the stress and treating it.
- Wellness is an active process of becoming aware of one's health, making choices to improve it, and taking actions toward a more balanced existence.

> • Not all stress management strategies work for everyone. For optimal results, treatment needs to be individualized for each person.

S tress Management is the new buzzword, and everyone even remotely associated with headache, whether it is the suffering person or the medical practitioner treating the headache, understands that stress needs to be controlled. Those of us who are sensitive to stress get this constant advice from our loved ones: "You need to control your stress better!" They think that by telling us this, the stress will disappear. Stress actually is a simple concept, but because of its myriad manifestations, it can become unnecessarily complex. It is important to understand stress, and then to take a practical approach to minimizing it. The methods discussed in this chapter are simple to employ and can be personalized to each individual's unique situation.

Some of you may experience headache only at times of stress, while others may experience improvement in their headaches at the time of their greatest challenges. Sometimes people experience headaches in the period following the stress when they are supposedly relaxing, such as on the weekends or during a vacation. However, did you know that headaches can cause stress? Sometimes the stress caused by the headache results in the next headache, creating a vicious cycle that is self-perpetuating.

"I Don't Have Stress"

Many people think that if they are happy with their jobs, have no significant problems with their families, or they do not have any pressures in life, they are not really stressed. Let us examine whether that is true or not. Stress can be experienced at the conscious level and at the subconscious level. Therefore, it is important to be aware of your own level of stress. As we learned in Chapter 19, headache is a symptom of some process gone awry in the body; it is the body's way of signaling a problem. It is important to stop and think of whether you are under stress or not, and whether you are taking the time to rejuvenate your body and mind.

Another misconception people have is that since their headache is triggered by a change in their internal or external environment—in response to a trigger such as chocolate or a change in the weather, for example—then stress-reduction strategies are not helpful. The fact is that when you strengthen your basic inner constitution, it raises the threshold at which your body creates a headache. When you do take the time to relax, you will realize just how much of an effect this unrecognized stress has on your life.

Equally important to the presence of a stressor is the *perception* of stress by an individual. How you respond to stress is more important than the actual stressful event. Dr. Dharma Singh Khalsa, a renowned physician specializing in pain management and anti-aging medicine, has created a version of the Stress Index called the Brain Longevity Stress Impact Scale, which incorporates your perception of the impact of the stressor, since each person responds differently to the same stressors. We have found this scale to be particularly useful in assessing how stress may be affecting people's lives. Before we go any further, it might be helpful for you to rate your level of stress in the stress index given below. In this index, a multiplier reflects your own perception of the effects of the stressor on you. This multiplier is on a scale from one to ten, based on how much stress you felt (or are still feeling) from the stressor. If a particular stressor did not bother you too much, you might multiply the stressor rating by two or three. However, if the stressor *devastated* you, you should multiply it by nine or ten. Please rate the stressors occurring within the last twenty-four months. If a particular stressor does not apply to you, score zero for that item.

See Stress Impact Index.

Brain Longevity Stress Impact Index

Event	Stressor Rating	Personal Perception Multiplier (1-10)	Score
Death of your child	100	_____	_____
Death of your spouse	99	_____	_____
Life-threatening illness	95	_____	_____
Prison term	80	_____	_____
Divorce	78	_____	_____
Marital separation	68	_____	_____
Death of a parent or sibling	68	_____	_____
Fired from your job	65	_____	_____
Pregnancy	60	_____	_____
Hospitalization for serious illness	58	_____	_____
Marriage	57	_____	_____
Foreclosure on a mortgage	57	_____	_____
Serious illness in the family	55	_____	_____
Birth of a child	50	_____	_____
Demotion at work	50	_____	_____
Lawsuit against you	50	_____	_____
Retirement	49	_____	_____
Sexual problems	45	_____	_____
Laid off from work	43	_____	_____
Problems with boss	40	_____	_____
Major business change	40	_____	_____
Major change in finances	39	_____	_____
Move to a new town	38	_____	_____
Death of a close friend	38	_____	_____

Career change	38	___	___
Change in frequency of arguments with spouse	35	___	___
Change in sleep habits	31	___	___
Problems with co-workers	30	___	___
Assuming a mortgage payment of more than 25 percent of your net earnings	29	___	___
Birth of first grandchild	28	___	___
Children leaving home	27	___	___
Problems with extended family	25	___	___
Significant lifestyle change	24	___	___
Illness for more than one week	23	___	___
Promotion at work	23	___	___
Change in political or religious beliefs	20	___	___
Assuming a mortgage payment of more than 20 percent of your net earnings	18	___	___
Change in social life	17	___	___
Change in diet	15	___	___
Vacation	10	___	___
Minor legal problem	10	___	___
Total Score			___

Interpretation of scores

If your score is:

Under 500:	you are relatively free from stress
Between 500 to 1000:	a state of low stress
Between 1000 to 2000:	a state of moderate stress
Between 2000 to 3000:	a state of high stress
Over 3000:	a danger zone

A prudent approach would be to start taking corrective actions if your scores are more than 2000. If you have a high score on this index, it means that you are engaging your stress response. Let us talk about this stress response, also known as the fight-or-flight response.

The Fight-or-Flight Response

Stress management is of paramount importance in the treatment of all types of headache. Today's work environments and family life are rapidly changing. It is becoming increasingly difficult to juggle the five important areas of an individual's life: work, family, society, finances, and recreation. Because of the lack of balance across these major spheres of life, people are experiencing greater stress than they can recall in recent memory.

The presence of a stressful event produces a cascade of physiological changes that ultimately leads to a state of hyper-vigilance. This state has many beneficial effects, primarily those having to do with survival. For example, when you perceive a threat, the body prepares you for addressing the threat with what is known as the fight-or-flight response. This response is our body's primitive, automatic, inborn response that prepares the body to fight or flee from perceived attack, harm, or threat to our survival. This is an acute response, and is beneficial only when it remains acute, and resolves when the perceived threat is over. For example, if you come face to face with a tiger, you need to either fight or run away, depending on which course will help you survive.

This stress response is primarily driven by adrenaline (also known as epinephrine), a hormone produced by the adrenal glands. When your brain perceives a threat, it starts a cascade of events, which activates the thinking part of your brain (known as the neocortex) and the emotional part of the brain (known as the limbic system). This registers as fear, which is then transmitted to other areas in the brain, resulting in the secretion of a hormone that activates the adrenal glands to produce adrenaline, cortisol, and other hormones. These hormones immediately affect the different organ systems to prepare the body to fight or run away. Some of these effects are:

1. Raising your blood pressure by activating the heart
2. Raising blood sugar by stimulating the liver, fat, and muscles to provide more energy
3. Causing blood vessels to constrict in order to speed the flow of blood
4. Slowing the metabolic functions that are not helpful in the stress response, such as digestion, sex drive, and fertility
5. Activating the brain so that you are hyper-alert and aware of what is going on around you.

Up to a point, all these are good effects. This is a very powerful mechanism designed to save your life. However, the type of stress you normally face in your daily life is not one of immediate threat to your safety or wellbeing. If it is not controlled, constant activation of the stress response can wreak havoc on your health, especially on your heart and brain. If the stress response is continually activated, day after day, your brain literally is bathed with cortisol, which has a devastating effect.

Most of the stressful events we encounter today are not a threat to our physical survival. Today's stressors consist of getting up in the morning, navigating rush-hour traffic, dealing with too much pressure at work, missing a deadline, making enough money to pay the bills, or having an argument with your boss or spouse. In fact, there are more neurological stressors these days than there were in the past; some never existed before. For example, the daily bombardment of information that our brain is subjected to adds stress to our lives, information from sources such as news, radio and television programs, movies, books, magazines, and, yes, even advertisements. The aptly named Mega-Information Syndrome is wreaking havoc on our brains. If you doubt the veracity of this, go spend a few days in solitude in the woods and experience the difference it makes in your nervous system. I have experienced this first hand. For someone who engages in stress management exercises routinely, my creativity has only expressed itself on occasions when I have taken time off from the normal routine of life and gone into the woods. I have written very few instances of poetry, but all of them were written when I've spent time with myself away from the information-loaded society. My creativity expressed itself without any effort on my part.

Besides the information overload, the technology at our fingertips adds its share of stress on the nervous system. How many minutes in a day are you totally free from the assault of technology in the form of telephones, smart phones, faxes, computers, personal data assistants (PDAs), television, voicemail, stereos, CD players, tablet devices, e-readers, and laptops? All of this electronic noise places an enormous burden on the nervous system, resulting in the periodic secretion of stress hormones.

We are not implying that life was necessarily better before the advent of these modern-day conveniences. However, the constant bombardment of information and the daily chores performed amid this fast-paced environment among the multitude of other responsibilities creates more stress on the brain and more resultant headaches, among other things. This stress only gets worse as we get older. One of the most worrisome consequences of this stress is the premature burnout of the nervous system, leading to, among other things, an increased incidence of dementia and other devastating neuro-degenerative conditions.

In short, most of the time, stress has to do with issues concerning our survival—not necessarily life-or-death survival, but survival nonetheless. If this daily stress is not conquered appropriately, then you might end up wishing you had been eaten by the tiger instead of suffering through all the diseases that stress has produced in your life. These stressors trigger the activation of our fight-or-flight response as if our physical survival was threatened. The stress hormones produced by our bodies for events that pose no real threat to our physical survival are toxic nonetheless.

Consequences of Negative Stress

According to research done at Stanford University in Palo Alto, California, stress induces an elevated cortisol level, which destroys the optimal functioning of the brain in three ways. First, cortisol inhibits the utilization of blood sugar by the brain. You may have noticed that when you are under stress, you experience short-term memory deficits. When the cells of the hippocampus cannot use glucose, it becomes difficult to form short-term memories. Second, cortisol interferes with the function of the brain's neurotransmitters. You may have noticed that under stress, you cannot recall previous memories, and you have problems with concentration. This is why cortisol is also known as the concentration killer. Third, and most important, cortisol kills brain cells by producing molecules known as free radicals, which can have long-term effects on brain functioning. In short, stress can cause both short-term and long-term changes in the brain.

During the period of stress, when your sole aim is survival, it is almost impossible to cultivate positive attitudes and beliefs. If you were to perform a brain-wave test during this survival mode, you would find that your brain wave activity is very fast. Generally speaking, faster activity is associated with excessive emotion, such as anger, love, and hate. When emotion is high, intelligence is low. The faster the brain-wave activity, the less relaxed and the less able to think you are. Your consciousness is focused on fear, not love. Your rational mind is unable to make clear choices and to recognize the consequences of those choices.

The Stress Response

1. As stress builds up, the body produces the hormones epinephrine, also known as adrenaline, and norepinephrine.
2. In response, the body produces **cortisol**, which limits the adrenaline response.

3. Chronic stress keeps the cortisol level up in an attempt to reduce the adrenaline.

4. Treatment should be aimed at identifying the cause of the stress and treating that instead of trying to decrease the cortisol level

One of the major consequences of chronic stress is burnout, which is essentially an exhausted brain. When you become overwhelmed with excessive stress, your life becomes a series of short-term emergencies. You live from crisis to crisis, with no resolution of each stressful event. If this cycle continues, there is a cumulative buildup of stress hormones. This causes disruption in the normal functioning of various organs of the body, which, if not corrected within a reasonable period, can lead to a multitude of diseases, culminating in premature death. Stress is known to cause disorders of the autonomic nervous system (headache, irritable bowel syndrome, high blood pressure) and disorders of our hormonal and immune systems (susceptibility to infection, chronic fatigue, depression, and autoimmune diseases like rheumatoid arthritis, lupus, and allergies).

The US National Academy of Sciences estimates that 70 to 80 percent of all visits to the family doctor are now stress-related. It has been shown that people with migraine are affected by stress more profoundly than those who never experience migraine. In addition, the coexisting conditions such as anxiety, depression, and insomnia are worsened with increased stress.

Restoring Balance

In its natural state of homeostasis, our body maintains a balance of the functioning of the various organs of the body. Since it is apparent that disease occurs when the body is out of balance, which most often is induced by stress, it stands to reason that health can be obtained by restoring this balance. Balance implies that there are opposing forces in a state of equilibrium. In the brain, there is a balance of two opposing forces, the sympathetic and parasympathetic divisions of the autonomic nervous system. The sympathetic nervous system is the one activated during the fight-or-flight response, causing activation of all the processes needed for that purpose: increased heart rate, elevated blood pressure, rapid, shallow breathing, and sweating. Normal functioning of the homeostatic mechanism requires the subsequent activation of the parasympathetic nervous system when the stressful event has passed, resulting in relaxation. Prolonged activation of the sympathetic nervous system from stress results in the typical physical and emotional consequences.

Fortunately, this process can be halted at any time. The first step is recognizing the early warning signs. The symptoms of stress buildup are unique to the individual and can be physical, emotional, or psychological. Some of these symptoms are given in Table 1.

Table 1: Early warning signs of excessive stress buildup

Physical	Emotional or Psychological
Muscle Tension	Anxiety
Headache	Irritability
Upset Stomach	Poor Concentration
Racing Heartbeat	Depression
Deep Sighing	Hopelessness
Shallow Breathing	Frustration
Low Energy/Fatigue	Anger
Frequent Colds	Sadness
Increased Sensitivity To _____(Fill	Fear
in the Blank)	Memory Loss
Poor Eating Habits	

Stress can cause headache in different ways. The most common form of stress headache is TTH. Headache as a response to stress can also occur *after* the stress. For example, some of you may experience the headache on the weekend after a very stressful week. This is typical of migraine headache. Anticipation of stress can result in headaches as well. Over time, if the stress continues, the intensity and the frequency of the headaches can worsen.

Excess stress does not always show up as the feeling of being stressed. Some people have a predominantly physical response to stress, while others have predominantly psychological reactions. If you tend to have more of a physical response, the stress tends to affect primarily your body, and you generally cope with it through physical responses, such as pacing. Conversely, you may feel lots of emotional stress and have very few physical symptoms or signs in your body. If you respond mainly psychologically, the stress tends to affect primarily your mind, and you generally cope with it through mental or psychological responses, such as rationalization. The following quiz, adapted from Dr. Dharma's brain longevity program, will determine if you respond to stress physically or mentally.

Your Coping Style

Read the following and mark all that apply to complete the sentence.

When I encounter stress:

1. I get butterflies in my stomach. _____

2. I find it hard to concentrate. _____

3. My pulse rate increases. _____

4. I start to worry about things I cannot control. _____

5. I feel as if there is not enough time to solve my problems. _____

6. I feel warm, and frequently begin to sweat. _____

7. I get a burst of energy, but soon feel hungry and weak. _____

8. My mind races with thoughts. _____

9. I get depressed. _____

10. I develop intestinal problems, such as diarrhea. _____

11. I have trouble sleeping. _____

12. I get mental images of the worst things that could happen. _____

13. My feet get cold. _____

14. My sex drive declines. _____

15. I talk to myself about my options. _____

16. My body feels almost paralyzed.

17. I escape mentally by focusing on happy thoughts.

18. I relieve tension by pacing, jiggling my leg, or engaging in some other nervous habit.

19. I become coldly logical.

20. My hands tremble and I feel shaky.

Item numbers 1, 3, 6, 7, 10, 11, 13, 14, 16, 18, and 20 reveal primarily physical responses to stress. If you marked more than five out of these eleven, you have a strong tendency to react physically to stress.

From the discussion so far, it may seem as stress is all bad. However, this is not true. Stress is neither good nor bad. It is neither negative nor positive. So, if it is neither of those things, then what is stress? And how does it work?

What Is Stress?

At its very basic level, stress is only one thing: *It is our body's powerful mechanism for automatically producing the energy we need to take action*, physically or emotionally. We can interpret this as:

Stress = Energy

Every time you need energy—whether it is lifting a heavy object, getting out of bed in the morning, or leading a meeting—your stress level automatically goes up. What defines stress as good or bad is how we use the energy, and what satisfaction, or lack thereof, we get out of this expenditure of energy.

When we talk about stress and headache, their relationship is self-perpetuating. As stress accumulates, the stress hormones remain activated, and the autonomic nervous system remains on hyper-alert in the fight-or-flight mode. As a result, one's thinking changes for the worse. You start expecting negative results to such an extent that it is hard to imagine a positive outcome. The ongoing stress manifests itself in different ways. The muscles become tense, your breathing becomes shallow, you have difficulty relaxing, and the stress keeps accumulating. Eventually, physical problems develop. These consist of headaches, high blood pressure, anxiety, and pain elsewhere in the body. The more negative stress you experience, the more headaches you experience. If nothing is done to limit stress, serious health problems will develop, such as heart disease, cancer, and gastro-intestinal disorders.

In order to decrease the ill effects of negative stress, you need to shift your focus. There is a saying that *what you focus on expands*. If you focus on stress, what expands is stress (which generally means the negative effects of stress). So instead of focusing on the negative, and attempting to figure out how not to be stressed, what you need to focus on is the opposite, known generally as **wellness**. You need to determine how to create wellness in your body, mind, and spirit. This is a five-step process:

1. First, you need to **recognize** what wellness looks like for you as a unique person. This is very personal as wellness is different for different people.
2. Second, you need to **understand** how wellness grows, as well as what puts it at risk.
3. Third, you need to determine your deep, personal **motivations** for lasting success.
4. Fourth, you need to choose the best **methods** and **tools** for achieving your goals.
5. Fifth, you need to plan for and take **action**.

What Is Wellness?

There are many definitions of wellness. According to the National Wellness Institute, wellness is an active process of becoming aware of, making choices, and taking action toward a more successful existence. The key words here are becoming aware of, making choices, and taking action. Wellness is a systemic concept. The main reason people want to become involved with their wellness has to do with satisfaction. If you feel satisfied with the outcome of any action, you will continue to do it. If the outcome does not satisfy you, this will create the physical effects of negative stress. However, what brings satisfaction to you may be quite different from what brings satisfaction to someone else.

Does Stress Management Really Work?

Balance can be achieved two ways: either decrease the stress (decreased activation of the sympathetic system) or increase relaxation (activation of the parasympathetic system). In this modern era, where our knowledge of the stress response at the cellular level has increased our understanding of the role of various brain chemicals, such as serotonin, norepinephrine, and cortisol, it has become easy to resort to drugs that can affect these neurochemicals. The drugs are helpful, especially in the short-term, where they temporarily counteract the effects of stress by balancing these chemicals. But all this does is mask the symptoms. The real key is to create internal balance by activating the parasympathetic system.

We will discuss strategies to achieve optimal wellness and to restore this balance, but first we will examine whether these strategies actually work. In a twenty-year study of stress management techniques, Dr. Selye and the Canadian Institute of Stress addressed two primary questions:

1. Do any of the stress management and wellness techniques actually work?
2. Do certain techniques work better for some individuals than for others?

Researchers have found that the answer to both questions is yes. They monitored different physiological reactions as well as other parameters to assess the effectiveness of stress management techniques. The results of the stress management question, with some additional observations, are given in Appendix 5. They discovered five proven stress control strategies, which they named the **Five Vital Skills**:

1. Clarifying your personal values and daily satisfiers
2. Being able to relax at will, anywhere, any time
3. Developing rewarding relationships
4. High performance nutrition
5. Essential exercise

In answering the second question, it was found that if the treatment for a particular person was not individualized, giving the wrong treatment actually *increased* their stress instead of lowering it. Perhaps that is a reason that some common strategies, such as relaxation, seem ineffective to some individuals. Therefore, people who cannot slow down, are always fast-paced, are always on the go, and are perfectionists may actually worsen if you tell them to slow down and relax. Teaching them how to relax too early in their stress management strategy might actually be more anxiety provoking than healing. It is critically important to choose the right treatment from the outset; otherwise, there is a high chance of failure.

To help individualize treatment for you, the first step is to determine which of the following Stress Types describes your response to stress:

1. **The Speed Freaks**: These people tend to be borderline workaholics or perfectionists, giving 110 percent effort to everything they do, no matter how (un)important it is. They have rapid speech, interrupt others frequently, and experience periods of deep fatigue after a period of all-out effort.

2. **The Worrywarts**: People in this group have trouble turning off their thoughts. They worry constantly but never take any action; thus, they experience frequent anxiety and are slow to recover from high-stress situations.

3. **The Drifters**: This group of people cannot focus on one thing but tend to expend their energy across many options without completing any tasks, and often feel dissatisfied with their lives.

4. **The Loners**: These people have difficulty forming intimate relationships. They feel uncomfortable with others and are often unfulfilled in relationships. They feel alone in social events and often drop out or cancel at the last minute.

5. **The Basket Cases**: These people tend to be always in energy crises and feel unable to carry out their daily activities. They experience frequent fatigue as well as aches and pains all over their bodies.

6. **The Cliff Walkers**: These people have many medical problems and are disasters waiting to happen. They never exercise, drink excessively, have high blood pressure and other risk factors, fatigue easily, and yet they believe that nothing bad will ever happen to them.

Are you stressed out? You're not alone! Take the short quiz on the next page developed by the Canadian Institute of Stress. This quiz will also help determine your stress type.

Action Exercises

1. So, let us make it personal to you. What are *your* personal early warning signs that you are just plain exhausted and getting close to running on empty in your wellness gas tank?
2. Did you get any insights about your own level of stress from the Stress Impact Scale?
3. What is your Stress Type? How are you going to address it?

Your Personalized Stress Profile Test

Instructions: Write a number in the blank at the left of each statement based on the frequency scale provided.

How frequently has each of the following statements been true about you during the past year?

0	1	2	3	4	5	6	7	8	9	10

Never   Rarely   Infrequently   Occasionally   Frequently   Very frequently

_____1. I feel used up at the end of the day.

_____2. I wish I could be as happy as other people seem to be.

_____3. I try to do two or three things at once, rather than focusing on one thing at a time.

_____4. If I could stop worrying so much, I would accomplish a lot more.

_____5. I don't seem to get the same kind of lasting satisfaction that I used to from the time I spend with friends.

_____6. I feel low on energy, exhausted, tired, or unable to get things done.

_____7. I feel that many people see me as being a lot more successful than I really feel I am.

_____8. I tend to hold my feelings inside rather than expressing them openly.

_____9. When something difficult or stressful is coming up, I find myself thinking about all the ways things can go wrong for me.

_____10. I don't feel really close to or accepted by the people around me, both family and friends.

_____11. I tire quickly.

_____12. I feel that my leisure time and recreational life don't express the really creative side of me.

_____13. I tend to anticipate others in conversation (interrupting, finishing sentences for the other person) rather than listening well and letting the other person finish speaking.

_____14. Whenever I try to put a worrisome thought out of my mind, it comes right back.

_____15. I don't handle conflicts or disagreements with people as well as I'd like to.

_____16. I frequently get the flu or a cold.

_____17. The ways I organize and use my time aren't a very accurate reflection of my interests.

_____18. I get uneasy when I'm waiting.

_____19. Decisions are hard for me because I spend a lot of time wondering if I've thought of all the alternatives.

_____20. I feel I should be spending more time with my family.

Your Stress Level and Stress Type Score Sheet

Instructions:

1. In the numbered spaces below, enter the numerical scores and answers from the questionnaire.
2. Add the numbers across each of the five rows. The total score for each row becomes your score for that Stress Type.
3. Add up your five Stress-Type scores. Enter this grand total in the Stress Score space provided. This final number summarizes your *overall stress level.*

STRESS TYPE SCORE

Basket Case

| Items | 1 | 6 | 11 | 16 | = _____ |

Drifter

| Items | 2 | 7 | 12 | 17 | = _____ |

Speed Freak

| Items | 3 | 8 | 13 | 18 | = _____ |

Worrywart

| Items | 4 | 9 | 14 | 19 | = _____ |

Loner

| Items | 5 | 10 | 15 | 20 | = _____ |

My total STRESS SCORE = _____

CHAPTER 22
Stress Management:
Positive Mind Over Matter

- The basic breathing method for relaxation involves breathing slowly and deeply.
- Many other methods describe variations of this process including autogenic relaxation, progressive muscle relaxation, and transcendental meditation.
- Meditation reduces blood lactate, reduces chronic pain, increases the production of serotonin, and improves the three key indicators of aging: hearing ability, blood pressure, and vision.
- Medical meditation directly affects the body's physical milieu and consists of specific breathing patterns, postures, mantras, and mental focus.

Now that we have established that stress is an important cause of headache, how do you counter stress? In the previous chapter, we discussed the various ways a negative *mindset* can wreak havoc with your *matter*, the physical body. Now we will discuss the ways a positive mindset can improve the health of your body.

There are many different ways of reducing stress and improving the body's response to it. Some recent discoveries have helped in our understanding of the stress response. One study found that the physical effects of stress are greatly magnified when people feel as if they have no control over their lives. Another important recent discovery showed that letting go of stress can largely negate its physical effects. Moreover, experiments have proved that a social support system greatly reduces the physical effects of stress.

One of the most common-sense approaches to stress management is to reduce the number of stressors in your life, but that is easier said than done! However, just because it is difficult to change your life and reduce the number of stressors does not mean that you should not do it. In the previous chapter, we learned that one of the top vital elements in stress management was clarity of your values and goals. This very important and effective technique helps to reduce the number of stressors for a number of people. We at Beverly Hills Headache Institute have developed the **Stress and Headache Reduction Program (SHARP)**, which incorporates stress management as a vital tool in headache reduction.

There are two basic psychological techniques to prevent chronic stress. Employing these can help you avoid most of the damage caused by chronic and negative stress. The first is to learn coping skills. Specifically, three skills provide the greatest protection against the negative effects of stress: 1) taking control of the stressor, 2) developing a social support system, and 3) learning how to release stress.

The second psychological method to combat stress is to evoke the opposite of the stress response: **the relaxation response**. In this chapter, we will discuss the relaxation response and show you how to incorporate it into your daily life.

How Do You Relax?

From studies conducted at Boston's Beth Israel Hospital and the Harvard Medical School, we know that relaxation techniques such as meditation have many physical benefits. Not only do they decrease headaches, they also improve self-esteem, self-confidence, and the body's general energy level. Dr. Herbert Benson showed that a fully relaxed mind is creative, intuitive, vibrant, and intelligent. The normal and natural state of the mind is the fully relaxed mind. Of course, in today's fast-paced world, it has become almost impossible for most people to attain this fully relaxed mind.

It might be interesting to narrate one of my own experiences with stress. The year was 1979, and the place was New Delhi, India. I was only fourteen years old when my father experienced his first heart attack. He was in his mid-fifties. Medical services in India back then were not as advanced as they are today, and he remained in the waiting room of the emergency department of a major hospital for over twelve hours in a half-dead state before he was finally seen by a physician. His condition was so dire that he was rushed to the intensive care unit (ICU). My mother was told that he had suffered a major heart attack and might not survive. My mother did not give up hope and remained in high spirits, staying by his side throughout his ordeal. Well! He survived, against expectations.

My older brother, who had already immigrated to the United States and had become a cardiologist, finally convinced my parents and me to move to the US after my father's recuperation. In subsequent years, he suffered many physical problems, including a few more heart attacks, cardiac arrest, stroke, congestive heart failure, and other physical ailments that come with age. But he never gave in to his illnesses.

My father beat the odds against survival for many years. Most physicians were amazed at his spirit and exuberance. With his turban and flowing silver beard, an aura of spirituality and calmness surrounded him. None of his physicians questioned the fact that he had remarkable staying power, and they were frequently amazed at his recuperative resilience. He passed away at the age of eighty-five after having lived thirty more years after his initial heart attack from which he was not expected to survive.

I attribute his remarkable recovery from his myriad medical issues to his lifestyle, of which meditation was an integral part. He had been meditating ever since he had become a practicing member of the Sikh faith. My experience with my patients and my study on meditation as medicine has proven to me beyond any shadow of a doubt the effectiveness of meditation as an instrument in treating many diseases. I have also witnessed that not only does it help patients with various medical problems; it also enables healthy people to improve their physical, mental, emotional, and cognitive health. My father was a shining example of living a spiritually aware and fulfilled life.

Yoga and Meditation

Dr. Dharma S. Khalsa, in his book *Meditation as Medicine*, demonstrates how meditation elicits the relaxation response and brings about physiological changes in the body that counter the effects of stress—the mental and emotional effects, and more importantly, the physical effects as well. He demystifies the mystical aspects of meditation and makes it very practical and easy to incorporate into your daily life. According to yogic theory, headache occurs only in persons whose minds are restless all the time. Once calmness of mind is achieved, headaches diminish or disappear altogether. This applies not only to tension-type headaches, but also to migraine and other types of headaches. Reduction of mental and emotional stress is accompanied by a measurable significant reduction in frequency and severity of headaches.

There are various meditative relaxation methods, but in almost all cases, the basic technique involves the following:

1. Finding a quiet place
2. Sitting in a comfortable position
3. Consciously slowing your breathing

One of the critical elements of relaxation is learning how to breathe properly. In fact, you cannot relax deeply without learning this simple yet essential element.

Breathing:

Most people have very shallow breathing. Have you noticed whether you breathe deep or shallow? The main reason for shallow breathing is *physical tension*, primarily caused by stress. Shallow breathing causes further stress. Breathing correctly, also called conscious breathing, has many powerful, physiological healing effects:

1. Improves digestion
2. Tones the nervous system, including the peripheral nerves
3. Cleanses the lungs and prevents respiratory infections, including the common cold
4. Enhances mood and brings relief from pain, anger, and fear
5. Helps healing as it shifts you away from the fight-or-flight mode

The basic breathing technique of yoga (also known as *pranayama*) is given here. If you only learn this basic breathing exercise and practice it daily, it will help to greatly reduce your stress, and as a result, the intensity and frequency of your headaches.

A detailed description of the different forms of yoga breathing exercises is beyond the scope of this book. We will discuss the three aspects of pranayama that are important in our topic of stress management. These are *posture, movement,* and *mental focus*. Combining conscious breathing with the right posture and the right mental focus will allow you to achieve relaxation quicker and in a more effective manner.

The Basic Technique for Proper Breathing (Pranayama), Known as the Complete Breath

- Sit or stand erect.
- Inhale a long deep breath through both nostrils.
- Retain the breath for several seconds.
- Exhale very slowly, holding the chest in a firm position.
- After completely exhaling, relax the chest and abdomen.

Posture and Movement:

The main effect of the different postures of yoga is to enhance the flow of energy and to increase the circulation of blood. This helps to create flexibility and balance within the body. As we discussed earlier, illness is a result of imbalance.

This balance is critical in all areas of life. Flexibility and balance go together. The postures and movements of yoga, combined with meditation, create flexibility and balance, not only physically but emotionally and spiritually as well. Yoga helps to restore endocrine balance (the body's hormones), which is quite deranged when under stress. The postures also help to balance the meridian system of energy flow.

Mental Focus:

Meditation aligns your conscious thought processes with the emotional centers, creating relaxing brain waves.

Breathing with this simple method for fifteen to thirty minutes can be very therapeutic and relaxing. With practice, you can slow your breathing significantly, to approximately one breath per minute. Make it a habit to meditate every morning to obtain the best benefit.

Alternate Nostril Breathing (also known as Anulom Vilom)

This type of breathing is very useful in relieving your headaches over the long term. Two versions of the technique are very helpful for headache control. One is the Calming Alternate Nostril Breathing technique, and the other is the Energizing Alternate Nostril Breathing technique. Which method you use depends on who you are as a person. Ideally, the yoga therapist will determine whether you will respond better to one or the other, based on your circumstances. Use a timer and set it for two minutes. This way you can concentrate on the breathing and not worry about whether you have done enough or not. As you get experienced, you can increase the time to five minutes or even longer.

Calming Alternate Nostril Breathing:

This technique involves the following (we assume that you are sitting in a comfortable position before starting this technique):

1. Inhale deeply through both nostrils.
2. Close the right nostril with the thumb of the right hand.
3. Exhale completely through the left nostril.

4. At the end of the exhalation, let go of the right nostril.
5. Inhale deeply through both nostrils.
6. Close the left nostril with the middle finger of the right hand.
7. Exhale completely through the right nostril.
8. At the end of the exhalation, let go of the left nostril.
9. Repeat.

Energizing Alternate Nostril Breathing:
This technique involves the following:

1. Close the right nostril with the thumb of the right hand.
2. Inhale deeply through the left nostril.
3. At the end of the inhalation, let go of the right nostril.
4. Exhale completely through both nostrils.
5. Close the left nostril with the middle finger of the right hand.
6. Then inhale through the right nostril, taking a long deep breath.
7. At the end of the inhalation, let go of the left nostril.
8. Exhale completely through both nostrils.

Regular conditioning of the nervous system through daily practice of pranayama will help to reduce the frequency, intensity, and duration of headaches. In addition to the breathing exercises, there are certain yoga exercises (known as *asanas*) that help to control headaches. These will be discussed in the chapter on exercise.

Which is right for you?
- Autogenic relaxation
- Progressive muscle relaxation
- Yoga
- Meditation
- Biofeedback
- Deep breathing
- Massage

Many other methods describe variations of this basic breathing process including autogenic relaxation, progressive muscle relaxation, and transcendental meditation. Learn the technique that works best for you. Practice the techniques whenever you feel yourself getting tense or stressed. It is a fact that simply becoming aware of your breathing and slowing it consciously can itself lower your stress level.

Autogenic Relaxation

The word autogenic means self-directed. This technique combines relaxation with two equally important processes: affirmation and visualization. A form of self-hypnosis, it utilizes breathing and focusing techniques to enter into a trance-like hypnotic state. *It is one of the most effective techniques for achieving a physically relaxed and mentally alert state.* Special audio programs have been designed to listen to while sitting in a comfortable position to guide you to a state of relaxation. Once you reach a deeply relaxed state, you can program your brain with positive affirmations and visualizations.

> **Autogenic relaxation** is a form of autohypnosis effective for treating a variety of ailments related to stress, including TTH and migraines. It decreases anxiety, depression, and fatigue, and increases your body's resistance to the negative effects of stress.

Affirmations are words or phrases that declare the positive values you want to ingrain in your subconscious and conscious mind. These can be phrases such as, "I am an excellent money manager," or "I am a confident person." Affirmations always start with "I" and always use positive words instead of negative ones.

Visualization is mental imagery, where you picture yourself doing whatever behavior you want to inculcate. The brain perceives mental pictures as actual events. For example, it has been shown in studies of participants of weight loss programs that people who were successful in losing weight and keeping it off were those who had a clear mental picture of what they would look like once they had lost the weight. The clearer the mental picture prior to starting the program, the more successful they were in achieving the goal.

Medical Meditation

Medical meditation combines yoga and meditation, and as such is a powerful countermeasure against the stress response. Medical Meditation is defined as the *use of advanced meditative techniques in a modern clinical setting.* It directly affects the body's physical milieu. It consists of specific breathing patterns, postures, mantras, and mental focus. In as little as three minutes, blood circulation improves, and the brain waves slow into the alpha frequency and even lower, making you more relaxed. Within approximately thirty minutes, your energy reaches a balanced state, which allows the body's healing powers to work.

Meditation has important physiological benefits. It has been shown to reduce blood lactate (a marker of stress and anxiety), reduce chronic pain significantly, increase the production of serotonin (which is critical in many conditions, including headaches and depression), and improve the three key indicators of aging: hearing ability, blood pressure, and vision.

Progressive Muscle Relaxation

Dr. Edmund Jacobson developed the progressive muscle relaxation technique more than fifty years ago. It is one of the most frequently used relaxation techniques in the world. It involves sequential tightening and releasing of all the skeletal muscles in your body. Using this technique, you isolate one muscle group, create a tension in that muscle group for five to ten seconds, and then let the muscle relax. This process is repeated in the next muscle group. Proponents of this technique state that it is guaranteed to produce relaxation as it is based on the physiology of the muscle. Whenever you release tension after creating it, the muscle relaxes. In fact, this process not only brings the muscle to its pre-tensed state; it actually relaxes the muscle further. Therefore, sequentially tensing and relaxing all the major muscle groups eventually relaxes the whole body.

Biofeedback

Biofeedback is a technique by which people are taught to induce their relaxation response by controlling certain physiological functions, such as heart rate, blood pressure, skin temperature, and muscle tension. These functions are normally under the control of the autonomic nervous system, which is, for the most part, involuntary. It was long thought that these functions were beyond voluntary control, but that has been proven wrong.

Chances are that you have already used biofeedback yourself. When you take your temperature using a thermometer or weigh yourself on a scale, you are receiving feedback about your body's condition. Once you have this information, you can take steps to improve the condition. Biofeedback machines are monitoring devices that give information in a similar manner. These machines can detect your internal bodily functions with great precision. The biofeedback machine allows you to see or hear the activity inside your body. Different types of machines assess different physiological parameters. One type of machine, for example, picks up electrical signals in the muscles, known as the electromyogram (EMG). It translates these signals into a form that you can detect, such as a flashing light bulb every time your muscles tense. If you want to relax the tense muscles, you have to try to slow down the flashing light bulb. Relaxation is a key component in biofeedback, especially when stress is a contributing factor in your condition.

The primary goal is to provide you with a tool that you can use to stop and/or prevent headaches. We hope that once you learn how to relax the muscles and control the headaches, you will not need the machines anymore. The temperature and EMG machines have shown effectiveness in treating both migraine and TTH.

Biofeedback can help in the treatment of many diseases and conditions. You need to recognize that certain conditions are under your control. You need to commit yourself to practicing biofeedback or relaxation exercises every day.

Discover the technique that works best for you. I suggest that you start with the basic breathing/relaxation technique described above, and then as you become more comfortable with it, feel free to experiment with the more advanced techniques. It is best to learn at least two or three different techniques that you can use depending on your circumstances. Some techniques are good for quick relaxation, and some are better for deep relaxation. The best time to relax is in the morning, but you can practice the techniques at any time during the day whenever you feel yourself getting tense or stressed.

You can choose the meditation technique that works for you. However, what is important is that *any* technique that reduces your stress is a valuable tool in your headache management program. Just choose a technique that works for you and get started, and remember to practice it daily.

Action Exercises

1. Begin a program of conscious relaxation by spending five minutes every morning doing deep breathing exercises.

2. Slowly increase the time and create a daily habit. Do at least five minutes of deep breathing every day.

3. Find a yoga studio in your area or call Beverly Hills Headache Institute for more information regarding yoga classes.

CHAPTER 23
Exercise and Headache Management

- Exercise consists of both physical exercise and mind-body exercise.
- Regular exercise lowers the incidence of headaches.
- Exercise can be very helpful in stopping headaches even in an acute migraine attack.
- The best preventative therapies for chronic headaches are mind-body exercises as well as aerobic exercise.
- There are specific mind-body exercises for headache treatment and prevention.

E xercise! The word itself conjures up images of rows and rows of daunting machines in the health club, with fitness buffs sweating and straining in their exercise clothes designed to show off their bulging muscles and toned physiques. Or it may bring up images of runners huffing and puffing on the treadmills or along the sidewalks. Or it may simply be images of people taking a leisurely stroll in the neighborhood park. But hardly anyone will bring up an image of a yoga class, with participants sitting in half-lotus positions with eyes closed and breathing deeply but in a relaxed state. That is not exercise! Or is it?

Exercise has long been known to be an effective strategy in improving many health conditions, including headaches. Being in good physical condition protects against a multitude of medical problems. There is physical exercise as well as mind-body exercise. If physical symptoms are caused by psychological and emotional issues, it stands to reason that any treatment strategy should include the treatment of the underlying issues as well. As we saw in previous chapters, repression of emotions can be an important cause of many chronic and degenerative conditions. For example, repressed anger has been shown to result in chronic headaches. Exercise is an effective method for relieving the mental and emotional pressures that can build up over time.

It is a well-established fact that regular exercise lowers the incidence of headaches, which makes it an important part of any treatment program. It is vitally important that you engage in some type of aerobic and anaerobic exercise.

Exercise has a tremendous impact on your brain. It keeps the brain younger by supplying it with growth factors that physically change the brain by increasing its size and increasing the number of connections among brain cells. The most important effect of exercise on the brain has to do with neuronal metabolism, the function of the nerve cells. Exercise increases the amount of oxygen and glucose to the brain, affecting the various neurotransmitters such as norepinephrine and cortisol, neuropeptides such as endorphins, and other critical functions. This induces creativity, intelligence, and memory.

We have seen how all these actions have a direct impact on headache. The effects of exercise in reducing stress are equally important regardless of whether you have primarily physical or psychological reactions to stress. People who are not physically fit exhibit a more heightened response to stress. In addition, exercise enhances mood by releasing endorphins, the body's own feel-good neuropeptides, creating a sense of tranquility. Exercise will not cure your headaches, but it will reduce their frequency and severity.

It has been shown that simply walking thirty minutes a day is enough to experience physical and mental fitness. Various studies have shown that it reduces mortality from heart disease. The type of activity you do is not as critical as many believe. What is more important is to find an activity you enjoy doing and do it regularly. If an activity is not fun, it will not be as effective in decreasing your stress.

Physical Exercise

Physical exercise ranges anywhere from simply walking for fifteen to thirty minutes three times per week to engaging in full-blown Mr. Universe contests. A discussion of different types of physical exercises is beyond the scope of this book. We will address general concepts and provide an overview of how exercise can be an effective part of your headache-relieving strategy.

Exercise, especially aerobic, can be particularly helpful in reducing stress as well as many stress-related conditions, such as headache. Aerobic fitness translates to efficient use of stress energy. Vigorous physical activity also helps you to unwind, which makes it particularly beneficial at the end of a high-stress day.

Stress results in the accumulation of toxic byproducts of metabolism, such as lactic acid. These acids build up in the muscles of the scalp in TTH, causing your head to feel heavy and your energy level to become low. Aerobic exercise stimulates the production of the neurotransmitter norepinephrine, which helps in reducing both anxiety and depression. As anxiety and depression improve, stress is reduced.

In addition, exercise stretches and relaxes muscles, which is helpful in preventing headaches. Regular aerobic and other cardiovascular exercise has been shown to reduce the frequency of both tension and migraine headaches by approximately 50 percent. All types of headaches benefit from exercise, although for most people, it is nearly impossible to engage in any type of physical activity during the acute migraine attack. However, paradoxically, exercise can itself be a trigger for migraine (known as exertional migraine). This usually occurs if you engage in strenuous physical exercise suddenly, without a period of gradual warming up. This causes blood vessels to dilate quickly to provide extra blood to the exercising muscles without giving them a chance to relax.

Physical fitness is a balance of three elements: **strength**, **stamina,** and **flexibility**. All three are important aspects of physical fitness. However, the measure of your fitness is subjective. It can best be ascertained by answering the following questions: Are you physically fit to do what you want and need your body to do, and still have energy left in reserve? Do you have the energy to complete your daily activities, including any normal crises, without undue strain on your health?

Acute therapy:

Exercise can be very helpful in stopping headaches, including tension and migraine headaches. For tension headaches, exercise should focus on stretching the tight muscles, especially in the neck, shoulders, and back.

In our experience, physical exercise can be very beneficial even during an acute migraine attack, provided it is performed in the first stage of the attack when the symptoms are not as severe and are manageable. During this stage, the blood vessels are still constricted, and exercise gently dilates them. The type of exercise during this type of headache should be aerobic, resulting in increased heart rate. Alternatively, mind-body exercises can be very beneficial in this stage, as we will discuss later in the chapter.

Preventative therapy:

Stress management is important both in acute treatment and in long-term prevention. Besides the techniques already mentioned in previous chapters, including the breathing exercises, the best preventative therapies for chronic headache are mind-body exercises as well as aerobic exercise. Aerobic exercise keeps the blood vessels flexible, reduces anxiety and depression, and reduces the perception of pain. Stretching and relaxing of the muscles results in reducing muscular tension, which is very helpful in preventing headaches. Performing physical exercises *after* a tension headache will help to prevent subsequent headaches.

Massage therapy

Massage therspy has been found to be very effective in preventing tension headaches by relieving muscle tension. Many cases of migraine headache are also triggered by stress and muscular tension; in such cases, massage therapy is very beneficial in relieving migraine headaches.

Mind-Body Exercises (Yoga)

There is a growing body of evidence that the majority of pain syndromes are psychologically induced. Mind-body exercises are extremely helpful in reducing stress, but equally important is their role in stimulating serotonin production. If you perform these exercises on a regular basis, you will see a reduction in the intensity, frequency, and duration of the headaches, until eventually, the headaches will cease completely. These exercises increase blood circulation to the brain. In tension headaches, the muscles in your neck, shoulders, and head are contracting to produce tightness and stiffness. Many yoga poses relieve tension and stress in the muscles of the neck, shoulders, and upper back. Any pose that involves hanging the head loosely is helpful. In addition, stretching the muscles of the neck and shoulders can work very well for headache relief, especially if it is done as part of a routine yoga practice.

We recommend that you consult an experienced yoga professional, such as a yoga therapist, before embarking on a yoga program. Some yoga poses may not be beneficial for your headache and may actually cause harm if not done properly. Yoga therapists generally have a lot more experience and training in using yoga in different medical conditions than regular yoga instructors have.

Having said that, the following three simple yoga poses have been found to be helpful in improving headaches.

Legs-up-the-wall pose (viparita karani):

One of the best exercises for headache relief is known as *viparita karani*, also known as the legs-up-the-wall pose. It is important to do this pose properly, because improper posture or doing it carelessly may cause injury.

For this pose, you will need some type of a support such as one or two thick blankets or a round bolster:

1. Sit with your right thigh against the wall and your legs stretched out in front of you.

2. Take a deep breath and exhale, and in a smooth movement, lay your head and shoulders onto the floor as you swing your legs up onto the wall.

3. Lift up your buttocks and slide the blanket or bolster under your hips in such a manner that the buttocks hang slightly between the wall and the bolster. It may take a few trials before you get the hang of it.

4. Keep your legs straight and firm against the wall.

5. Lift your head up off the floor and put a towel under your neck so the spine is not lying flat on the floor.

6. Stay in this pose for ten to fifteen minutes and breathe gently but deeply. Close your eyes. Make sure you relax your muscles, especially of the face, neck, and jaw.

7. When you are ready to come out of the pose, gently lift your hips up by bending your knees and gently push against the wall with your feet. Remove the support, lower your pelvis to the floor, and gently slide your legs down the wall on one side.

8. Stay on your side for a few breaths and then gently come back up to a sitting position.

Forward-fold pose (Padahastasana):

1. Stand erect with legs together.

2. Inhale slowly and raise your arms out to your sides.

3. At the horizontal level, turn your palms upward.

4. Continue to inhale and move your arms upward until your biceps touch your ears.

5. Turn your palms forward.

6. Stretch your body up from the waist.

7. Keeping your lower back concave, exhale and bend forward until the trunk of your body is parallel to the ground; stretch out your shoulders at the horizontal plane and inhale.

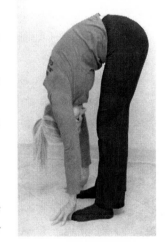

8. Exhale while bending down further until your palms rest flat on the ground and your chin touches your knees.

9. Maintain this posture for two to three minutes without bending your knees.

10. Inhale, come up slowly to the vertical position, and stretch your arms above your head.

11. Exhale, drop your arms, and turn your palms downward at the horizontal position.

12. Continue to exhale as you return to a normal standing position.

Half-wheel pose (Ardh-kati-chakra-asana):

1. While inhaling, slowly raise your right arm upward and out to your side.

2. At the horizontal level, turn your palm upward.

3. Continue to inhale deeply and raise your arm until your bicep touches your right ear, palm facing the left side.

4. Stretch your right arm up.

5. While exhaling, bend your trunk slowly to the left.

6. Your left palm slides down along your left thigh as far as possible.

7. Do not bend the right elbow or the knees.

8. Maintain for about a minute with normal breathing.

9. Slowly come back to a vertical position while inhaling.

10. Stretch the right arm up. Feel the pull along a straight line from the waist up to the fingers.

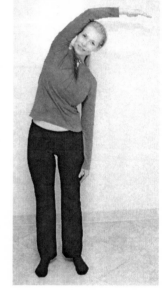

11. Bring the right arm down as you exhale to normal position.

12. Relax in a standing position.

13. Following these steps, perform the pose on the left side.

The best yoga therapy for your headache is one that is personalized for you based on factors such as the cause of your headache, your physical conditioning level, the presence of other medical or physical conditions, and other factors that are unique to you. You should try to find a qualified yoga therapist in your area who can personalize the yoga therapy for you.

Exercise Plan for Headache Control

1. Give your body the benefit of at least thirty minutes of physical exercise at least five days per week. Any type of aerobic exercise, whether it is walking, running, swimming, cycling, or aerobics, will be beneficial. The main idea is to get your body moving.

2. Include a few minutes of stretching before and after exercise.

3. Spend a few minutes every day in the three yoga poses shown above or as prescribed by a yoga therapist.

CHAPTER 24
Diet and Headache

- Nutritional therapy helps to repair the damage done to the brain by cortisol and other toxins, and prevents further damage.
- Excess sugar in your diet eventually is converted to fats.
- Limiting the amounts of saturated fat in your diet, combined with eating more complex carbohydrates or low GI foods, can be very helpful in treating and preventing your headaches.
- Lifestyle modification can provide significant relief from your headaches in as little as four weeks.

To sustain life all of us have to feed our bodies, but what we eat can make us healthier or sicker. There is an undeniable connection between what you eat and the occurrence (and recurrence) of headaches, especially migraine. This connection goes beyond just dietary triggers of headache. In this chapter, we will focus on diet and its relationship to headache. It has recently been shown that obesity is associated with more severe and frequent migraine attacks, chronic daily headache, and transformed migraine. We will examine some of the general principles governing diet and their relationship to the production as well as prevention and treatment of headache.

Nutritional therapy includes diet, natural medicinal tonics, and supplementation with specific nutrients. Nutritional therapy can begin with your next meal. Contrary to popular belief, results can be quick and dramatic. Nutritional therapy helps to repair the damage done to the brain by stress hormones and other toxins, and prevents further damage. Adequate nutrition supplies the brain cells with the building materials they need for proper functioning.

In order to live, the human body requires certain essential substances. These include *macronutrients* (carbohydrates, fats, and proteins) and *micronutrients* (vitamins and minerals). Most of these are obtained through our diet, and therefore, we are what we eat. When we eat healthy, nutritious food, we remain healthy; when we eat unhealthy, nutrition-poor food, this creates all sorts of diseases including headaches.

Diet-related diseases have become more common in the last century. The typical diet over a hundred years ago was much different from the prevalent diet in most industrialized societies today. Epidemiologic studies have shown that since 1910, consumption of fat has increased, especially the ratio of unsaturated-to-saturated fat. Consumption of complex carbohydrates has dropped from 37 percent to 21 percent, whereas the consumption of simple sugar has increased from 12 percent to 25 percent of the total diet. More than half of the standard American diet, which we term the *SAD diet*, consists of fat and sugar, which really is a sad thing. One of the consequences of this eating pattern is the increasing incidence of obesity.

Along with the increased consumption of fat and sugar, there has been a decrease in the consumption of healthy foods. More than half of all Americans consume no fruits or vegetables at all.

The far-ranging effects of this diet are all too obvious. The increase in heart disease, cancer, many degenerative diseases, and a whole host of other diseases has been attributed in large part to our lifestyle.

Carbohydrates

Carbohydrates are the staple of most diets and comprise sugars, starches, and fiber. In fact, the basic building block of carbohydrates is the sugar molecule. A simple classification of carbohydrates, which will help in our understanding of their metabolism, is to divide them into two major groups:

1. **Simple** carbohydrates are sugars such as fruit sugar (fructose), corn or grape sugar (dextrose or glucose), and table sugar (sucrose). Simple sugars are easy to identify by their sweet taste.
2. **Complex** carbohydrates are compounds made from three or more linked sugars. Our digestive system breaks down most carbohydrates into simple sugars, specifically glucose. Starches and fibers are essentially chains of sugars linked together. Complex carbohydrates are not sweet.

Simple sugars are digested easily and absorbed rapidly into the bloodstream, causing a rapid rise in blood glucose levels. Complex carbohydrates are broken down slowly and do not result in the high peaks of blood glucose levels seen with simple sugars.

How the Body Processes Sugar

Let us examine the relationship of fat to sugar in the diet. Excess sugar from diet is converted to fats. There are many types of sugar; however, all the different types are broken down into glucose. When blood sugar rises, the body produces the hormone insulin, which helps to metabolize the sugar and return it to normal levels within the body. Insulin also helps metabolize the fat in blood.

White sugar is nothing but sucrose in a highly concentrated form without any nutritional value. (The addition of various chemicals to crystallize the sugar removes all proteins, minerals, vitamins, and other substances.) Sucrose is broken down into glucose in the intestines and absorbed quickly into the bloodstream. The sudden increase in blood sugar results in a compensatory rise in the amount of insulin released into the bloodstream to counteract the high levels of sugar. Insulin facilitates entry of glucose into other organs. This lowers the blood sugar quickly. This also results in lowering the levels of serotonin, which can result in a headache.

Insulin Resistance

The muscles and other tissues only take up as much glucose as they need and the rest is stored in the liver as glycogen. But there is a limit to how much glycogen can be stored. When this limit is reached, insulin stimulates the liver cells to convert the excess sugar into fat. The high amount of insulin secreted overshoots the mark and causes the blood sugar to become too low. This causes a yo-yo effect on the blood sugar levels: **hyperglycemia** (high blood sugar) alternating with **hypoglycemia** (low blood sugar). Hypoglycemia, in turn, causes the blood fat levels to rise, and causes the release of epinephrine, which increase aggregation of platelets, thereby worsening the effect on headaches. These higher peaks and lower troughs of blood glucose eventually lead to **insulin resistance**, which means the cells do not respond to insulin, causing both blood sugar and insulin levels to stay high. Excess fat (obesity) and lack of exercise also lead to insulin resistance. Data from the *Insulin Resistance Atherosclerosis Study* suggests that cutting back on refined grains and eating more whole grains can improve insulin sensitivity.

Glycemic Index

Another way of classifying carbohydrates is to determine the **Glycemic Index**. This index measures how fast and how much the blood sugar rises after ingesting a particular food. Foods with a **high** GI are absorbed quickly and cause a quick and strong rise in blood glucose levels. Most of the simple carbohydrates belong to this group. These foods have been linked with diseases such as diabetes, heart disease, stroke, and obesity. The factor that determines a food's GI is how highly processed the carbohydrates are. **The more processed the sugar, the higher the GI, the quicker it gets absorbed, and the greater the probability of it being converted into fat.**

Other factors influence how quickly blood sugar can be raised by carbohydrates:

1. **Fiber content:** Fiber protects the carbohydrates from immediate and rapid attack by digestive enzymes. This slows the release of sugar molecules into the bloodstream.
2. **Ripeness:** Ripe fruits and vegetables tend to have more sugar than unripe ones, which increases the GI.
3. **Type of starch:** Starch comes in many different forms. Some starches are easier to break into sugar molecules than others.
4. **Fat content:.** The presence of fat slows the conversion of carbohydrates into sugar, which in turn slows the absorption of carbohydrates into the bloodstream.
5. **Physical form:** Finely ground grain is more rapidly digested than coarsely ground grain. This is one of the reasons white flour has a higher GI than whole-wheat flour.

Glycemic Load

The classification of carbohydrates can get even more involved. The glycemic index alone does not tell us everything we need to know about food's impact on blood sugar levels. For example, a given food's GI does not tell us anything about the amount of carbohydrate in it. A new classification takes into account both the amount of carbohydrate in the food and the impact of that carbohydrate on blood sugar levels. This measure is called the **glycemic load** (GL). A food's glycemic load is determined by multiplying its glycemic index by the amount of carbohydrate it contains. Foods are divided into those having low, medium, or high GL. However, for our purposes, we need only to understand the changes in diet that will be beneficial to us.

Adding Good Carbohydrates Helps Prevent Headaches

Let us relate all this information together to see how carbohydrates can help in the prevention of headaches. One important factor in headache prevention is the management of serotonin levels in conjunction with the regulation of blood sugar and insulin levels. Consuming complex carbohydrates does not result in high peaks and low troughs in the blood sugar and insulin levels, and serotonin is maintained at a steady level, which prevents headaches as well as depression and anxiety.

A diet high in fats and refined sugar is directly implicated in causing headaches. To prevent headaches, start by replacing simple with complex carbohydrates. Most of the calories should come from carbohydrate sources such as fruits, vegetables, and grains. The table below lists some examples of good carbohydrates. Not only will these foods help protect you against a range of chronic diseases; they will also decrease the impact of your migraine headaches.

Good carbohydrates	Bad carbohydrates
Fruits Vegetables Whole wheat bread Brown rice Whole grain pasta Whole oats	Snacks made with refined sugars and white flour, such as cookies, ice cream, cakes, donuts, and candy—all those things that taste oh-so-sweet.

The bottom line is to replace highly processed grains, cereals, and sugars with whole-grain products.

Fats

We all need fat in our diet, but the amount of fat most of us consume is in excess of what our bodies require. In addition to the excess fat, eating the wrong type of fat has also been implicated in the production of migraine headaches. Let us briefly examine some important facts about fat and how you can modify your fat consumption to improve your headaches.

There are three main types of fats: *saturated, polyunsaturated,* and *monounsaturated.* High amounts of saturated fat in the blood are thought to promote clustering of platelets, which has been associated with lowering the levels of serotonin, resulting in headache.

The unsaturated fats are the good fats and include the *omega-3 fatty acids*. These omega-3 fats are helpful for headache patients, as they inhibit the clustering of platelets. Most of the omega-3 fatty acids are found in fish, especially fatty, cold-water fish such as salmon and mackerel. Vegetarian sources include flax seeds and flaxseed oils, soybeans, walnuts, and canola oil. A list of the different types of fats is given in Appendix 7.

Types of Fat

Saturated fats are mostly found in animal products, such as meats and dairy products, and some vegetable products. They raise blood cholesterol. They are solid at room temperature.

Polyunsaturated and **monounsaturated fats** are derived mainly from plants. They lower blood cholesterol. They are liquid at room temperatures.

Hydrogenation converts these fats into saturated fats as well as *trans fats*, making them solid at room temperature.

Trans fats are a particularly harmful unsaturated fat. Trans fats are generally present in small amounts in various animal products and are produced during hydrogenation. Trans fats are thought to be even more harmful than saturated fats because they can increase bad cholesterol and lower good cholesterol quite significantly.

Omega-3 Fatty Acids

Omega-3 fatty acids are derived from fish oils and some plant oils. The fish oils contain *docosahexanoic acid* (DHA) and *eicosapentanoic acid* (EPA), while the vegetable oils and walnuts contain *alpha-linolenic acid* (ALA).

Limiting the amounts of saturated fat in your diet and eating more complex carbohydrates or low GI foods can be very helpful in treating and preventing your headaches. Other dietary changes helpful for headache control include drinking plenty of fresh water, consuming vitamins, especially the B vitamins riboflavin (B2), niacin (B3), and pyridoxine (B6), vitamins C and A, and minerals such as magnesium and calcium.

Beyond Micro and Macronutrients

In terms of diet, most of the problems occur when you consume foods that have minimal nutritional value. Processed foods, whether they are refined sugar-containing foods or other junk foods such as potato chips, have a deleterious effect on the internal environment, affecting the nervous, endocrine, and immune systems. Constant bombardment of unhealthy foods saps the essential energy of the body, the energy needed to repair itself. Unnatural living habits and improper diet play a large role in creating the majority of the illnesses plaguing humankind today.

Let us now take a step backward into ancient civilizations and consider our diet from a different perspective. Just looking at the nutrient quality and the amount and type of fats, carbohydrates, proteins, vitamins, and minerals is not enough. The foods we consume have other properties that are not easily measured by modern scientific methods. Let us explore how the ancient Chinese and Indian cultures viewed food, and then let us discover what we can learn from them in order to improve our diet.

For ease of understanding, we can divide all foods into two groups:

- **Positive** foods are foods that are health promoting. All the positive foods contain a lot of fiber and are thus lighter and easier to digest. These foods include fruits and vegetables, and to a lesser extent, grains and cereals. Most of these foods are alkaline, and help to maintain the alkalinity of blood.
- **Negative** foods are health depleting. Negative foods are heavy in proteins, starches, fats, and sugars. They are harder to digest and often

are constipating. These foods are acidic in nature and thus promote ill health.

In order to reap the maximum health-promoting benefits, foods should be as fresh as possible. When freshness is lost, vitality of the food is lost as well.

Concept of Hot and Cold Foods

According to TCM, Ayurvedic medicine, and other Eastern traditions, food has an energy profile. Many people prefer eating organic (non-processed) foods. However, these supposedly healthy foods may not be as healthy as you think. Why is that?

Food exhibits organic energy just like other living beings. This energy can be classified as either hot or cold. Hot does not refer to the temperature of the food but rather to its energy profile. (See Food Energy Chart, Table 1). If you have too much heat in your body and you consume hot foods, your condition will worsen.

To illustrate this principle, let us consider an example. How many people do you know who are on a diet and eating only salads? How many of them are actually losing weight, not starving, and still getting enough nutrition? Besides the fact that they may be starving themselves and not getting enough micro and macronutrients in their diet, there is another reason why they may not be losing weight. The natural energy of most raw foods is **cold**, so if you have a cold constitution, which is hindering you from burning off all that you are eating, then eating salads is going to make things worse. (According to TCM, there are nine different types of body constitutions. The person with a cold and pale constitution is sensitive to cold, has a high tolerance of heat, and is noted to be an introvert and a quiet type of a person. Interested readers are encouraged to explore the energetic aspects of food and body constitutions further.).

The Ayurvedic Prescription

As we mentioned earlier, humans exist in three stages: Rajas, Tamas, and Satvik. According to Ayurvedic medicine, food can also be classified into three different grades known as rajasic, tamasic, or saatvik. These grades assess the quality of a food that goes beyond the gross quality of fats, proteins, and carbohydrates. This is the quality of the food's purity in terms of its effect on vitality and consciousness. Food is the carrier of the life force called prana:

1. **Rajasic foods**: Foods that are bitter, sour, salty, hot, harsh, or pungent are considered rajasic, and are the causes of diseases of the body and depression of the mind. These foods cause you to feel agitated and over-stimulated, leading to pain, misery, and sickness. These foods include meat, fish, and alcohol.

2. **Tamasic foods**: Foods that have lost their freshness over time and become stale, tasteless, and rotten. These foods can make you feel tired and sluggish. Overeating is a tamasic quality.

3. **Satvik foods**: Foods conducive to longevity, happiness, strength, and purity of body and mind as well as freedom from disease. These foods produce calmness, alertness, vitality, and the feeling of freshness. Satvik food consists of lightly cooked vegetables with minimal spices, fruits, nuts, honey, milk and milk products, butter, and grains.

The Ayurvedic diet prescription is the satvik diet, as this promotes health, strength, energy, and courage, but more importantly, it provides subtle nourishment for the purity of consciousness. Satvik foods are fresh and freshly prepared foods. They are light, easy to digest, and refreshing.

According to this philosophy, people prefer to eat according to which stage of life they are in. So, if you are a satvik person, you will prefer to eat satvik foods.

One important belief of Eastern medicine is that just as food affects your mind, your thoughts and emotions affect your food. Even the most nutritious food, if eaten in a state of anger, will not provide optimal nutrition.

Space does not permit us to delve too deeply into this philosophy of diet and nutrition, and the disease producing or health promoting effects of various foods. We encourage you to learn more about these principles and to change your diet accordingly.

This lifestyle modification produces relatively quick results. You do not have to wait thirty years to see the benefits of changing your lifestyle.

In as little as four weeks, you will experience significant relief from your headaches, whether a diminishment in the level and severity of pain or a reduction in the number of headaches. Lifestyle modification does not give as quick a result as a painkiller in alleviating your headaches, but it will help you develop good habits that you can use for the rest of your life, which will relieve you from dependence on medication and help you to achieve freedom from headaches.

The Headache Prevention Diet

The headache prevention diet is not really a diet, but a set of principles. Instead of counting calories, incorporate these easy-to-follow principles in your diet:

1. **Eat a balanced diet**. First of all, throw away the food pyramid. A balanced diet means a balance of whole grains, fruits, vegetables, and protein (preferably non-animal based). Approximately half of your diet should contain a wide variety of different types of whole grains. Another 25 percent of your diet should consist of fruits and vegetables. The majority of the protein should be from non-meat sources such as soy, yogurt, cottage cheese, almonds, and grains. Virtually all meat is high in fat. Even the leanest chicken contains more fat than any of the non-meat protein sources. Eat more positive foods and limit the amount of negative foods.

2. **Eat a low bad-fat diet**. You have already seen how fat can cause headaches, among other things. Avoid hydrogenated or partially hydrogenated oils at all costs. Margarine and shortening are two examples of the fats that should be avoided. A 15 to 20 percent reduction in fat is highly advisable.

3. **Eat a nutrient-dense diet**. Avoid empty calories from simple carbohydrate snacks and carbonated beverages. Your brain requires many nutrients on a daily basis for optimal functioning.

4. **Eat regular meals**. Eating regular meals keeps blood glucose levels from becoming extremely low. Your brain requires a constant supply of

glucose for optimal functioning. The best way to avoid hypoglycemia is to eat a sensible diet rich in complex carbohydrates and proteins.

5. **Eat raw, unprocessed foods.** Processing of foods removes essential nutrients and adds various preservatives to prolong the shelf life. These preservatives and other chemicals, such as food colors, can trigger headaches. The more processed food you consume, the more headaches you will have.

6. **Drink plenty of water.** Water is the true elixir of life. Limit the amount of carbonated drinks you consume, whether they are regular or diet sodas.

7. **Take nutritional supplements.** In this day and age, it is virtually impossible to get optimal doses of all vitamins and minerals from diet alone. It is recommended that everyone take a good quality multivitamin and an omega-3 supplement at the least. Most people should also consume a B-complex vitamin supplement, especially as it can help in reducing headaches.

8. **Eat only when hungry and not to the extent of overeating.** Thoroughly chew your food so that the food is well mixed with the saliva, which contains digestive juices. The amount of saliva produced is in direct relationship to the amount of chewing. If there is inadequate chewing, the subsequent gastric and intestinal digestion is affected.

9. **Eat satvik foods.**

Action Exercises

1. List foods that you regularly consume at breakfast, lunch, and dinner.

2. List foods in the healthy diet mentioned in this chapter that you have consumed in the last week.

3. Prepare a balanced diet plan based on the discussions in this chapter.

CHAPTER 25

Nutraceuticals: Vitamins, Supplements, and Herbal Preparations

- Herbal supplements and vitamins are good alternatives to taking medications for the treatment of headache. However, they should be used with caution, as they can have side effects and may interfere with prescription and OTC medications.
- Butterbur, feverfew, riboflavin, and magnesium are some of the non-medication supplements that have been evaluated in studies for migraine prevention.
- Migrelief is a combination of feverfew, magnesium, and riboflavin, and has been found to be effective in preventing headaches.

I n the next few pages, we will discuss some of the vitamins, supplements, and herbal treatment approaches that have been proven effective in scientific studies comparable to the types of scrutiny performed on pharmaceutical drugs. The term *nutraceutical* is defined as "any substance that may be considered a food or part of a food and provides medical or health benefits." The general impression among the public is that all herbal and vitamin supplements can be taken safely. While this statement is true for the most part, you should use them with caution, as they can cause side effects and can interfere with other medications you may be taking. It is important that you discuss these with your physician in order to ensure that you do not have any contraindications to taking these herbs and other supplements. Most of these approaches are not designed for quick relief. They are generally used in preventing migraine headaches over the long term, and have to be taken for a period of days or weeks before you notice any improvement in the frequency, duration, and intensity of your headaches.

Coenzyme Q10 (CoQ10) and Vitamin B2 (Riboflavin)

CoQ10 and Vitamin B2 have been studied in prevention of migraine headaches. Both of these are known to improve the function of the mitochondria, the powerhouses of the cells in our bodies. Vitamin B2 is necessary for normal energy metabolism. It is found in milk, cheese, dark green leafy vegetables, organ meats, almonds, and whole grains. In one study, it was shown to markedly reduce the number of headaches in migraine patients. The difference, compared to placebo, was highly significant. The only side effects when taking Vitamin B2 were minor, consisting of diarrhea and increased urination. The dose of Vitamin B2 was 400 milligrams daily.

Similarly, CoQ10, at a dose of 100 milligrams three times daily, has shown substantial reduction in the headaches of patients who suffer migraines. According to Dr. Rozen, who was one of the authors of the study on CoQ10 published in *Cephalalgia*, the journal for the International Headache Society, "Coenzyme Q10 looks to be an excellent choice for initial therapy for prevention of episodic migraine if confirmed by controlled studies of efficacy. It can be given to almost any age group without fear of significant side effects." In medical practice, both these supplements are very good alternatives to standard medications. However, it is important to take the right dosage. Most CoQ10 preparations contain very minute amounts of the substance, usually in the 30-milligram range. In addition, as with other preventative medications, the effects of CoQ10 may not be noticeable until at least five to ten weeks of therapy.

CoQ10 may have other beneficial effects as well. It has been found to have useful effects in heart failure, stroke, cancer, aging, high blood pressure, and even AIDS. It is synthesized in the body through a very complex process, requiring seven different vitamins (six of them belong to the B-complex group, and vitamin C), and several trace elements. For migraine prevention, we recommend taking 300 milligrams daily. Although there is no scientific data, we believe the soft-gel capsules are better than tablets.

Butterbur (Petasites hybridus)

Butterbur is a plant-based herb that has been used medicinally for thousands of years. It has been prescribed in Germany for over thirty years, but has only recently been studied in the United States. It has two active ingredients, both of which have an anti-inflammatory effect. It also inhibits the production of histamine, which accounts for its beneficial effect on allergies. Recent scientific data have shown that this herb may be an effective preventative therapy for migraine headache at a dose of at least 50 milligrams twice daily. However, one study comparing 50 milligrams and 75 milligrams twice daily showed the higher dose to be more effective. It is well tolerated and does not have significant side effects. The major side effects noted were gastrointestinal (nausea, burping, and vomiting) and were mild.

Feverfew (Tanacetum parthenium)

This herb has been used for headache treatment for many years. It is a member of the sunflower family. The term *feverfew* is adapted from the Latin word *febrifugia* or *fever reducer*. It contains compounds known as *sesquiterpene lactones,* which inhibit platelet aggregation and the release of serotonin from platelets and other cells. Anecdotal evidence from Great Britain, where it has been used extensively, shows that more than 70 percent of patients feel substantially better after taking feverfew leaves. There have also been several well-designed studies evaluating the effectiveness of feverfew in preventing headaches. Most of the studies have shown positive results in headache relief as well as a decrease in the accompanying symptoms of nausea and vomiting. It is a good alternative for patients who have not improved using conventional therapies or who cannot tolerate standard medications due to side effects.

Magnesium

Magnesium is a mineral that is important in the normal functioning of the human body. It relaxes the central nervous system. Magnesium deficiency, the most common mineral deficiency, has been closely linked to migraine headaches. It is known that magnesium can cause constriction of blood vessels. One theory states that lack of magnesium causes the serotonin in the body to flow unchecked, which leads to narrowing of the blood vessels and releases pain-producing chemicals, such as substance P and prostaglandins. The recommended daily allowance (RDA) for magnesium is 420 milligrams for men and 320 milligrams for women, and most people do not get nearly as much from their diet. In addition, magnesium can be depleted from the body by such substances as caffeine and some medications. When you combine low intake of supplemental magnesium with high intake of food and medicines that deplete the magnesium in your body, this can lead to a magnesium-deficient state. Numerous studies have shown that magnesium supplementation can be helpful in treating migraine headaches.

Even if you do not have a magnesium deficiency, you will likely benefit from supplementing your diet with oral magnesium. The best way to optimize your magnesium levels is with magnesium found in whole foods. Green leafy vegetables such as spinach and Swiss chard, and nuts and seeds such as almonds, pumpkin seeds, and sunflower seeds are great sources of magnesium. When it comes to magnesium supplements, there are at least nine different types of supplements available. The one that has been used in scientific studies and shown to be beneficial for migraine patients was magnesium citrate. Side effects are minimal, especially if you don't take too high a dose. High doses can lead to diarrhea.

The manufacturers of a commonly found natural preparation have combined three of the substances discussed above, feverfew, magnesium, and riboflavin, in a single preparation known as **Migrelief**. It has been found to be particularly effective in preventing headaches, especially in patients who cannot or do not wish to take preventative medications for their recurrent headaches. Like with other natural treatments, the supplement has to be taken for at least a few weeks before you may notice any significant improvement in your headaches. Similarly, a different preparation, **Migravent**, combines four of the substances above: butterbur, Vitamin B2, magnesium, and CoQ10.

CHAPTER 26
Homeopathy

- Homeopathic medicine views headache in the context of the whole person: physical, emotional, mental, and social.
- The homeopathic approach to migraine and headache is to stimulate the individual's forces of recovery by aiming treatment at the root cause of the ailment rather than masking the pain with pain medications.
- The remedy is the actual diagnosis, because each remedy is selected according to the individual's unique set of symptoms.

H omeopathy (derived from the Greek words *homoion*, meaning similar, and *pathein*, meaning disease) is founded upon principles that are in turn derived from natural laws. It was discovered in 1796 by Dr. Samuel Hahnemann, a physician who had become disillusioned by the practice of medicine. It is a safe, scientific, and logical system for the treatment of disease. The basic premise of homeopathy is the principle of *similia similibus curantur*, which means *like cures like*, whereas allopathy (*allos* means different) operates on the principle that the symptoms of a disease are cured by a medicine that opposes the symptoms.

The homeopathic physician, when treating a patient, has the objective to diagnose, but not in the sense that a Western physician diagnoses the problem, wherein the diagnosis is used to guide his therapy. The approach to treatment underscores the basic difference between allopathic and homeopathic medicine. The first aim of allopathic medicine is to group patients according to their diagnoses, such as migraine headaches; the patients with the same disease will be treated with similar medications. For the homeopathic physician, the objective is to decipher the true symptoms of each individual patient, not the outward manifestation of the true symptoms. The treatment is based upon the patient as a whole rather than the similarity of his symptoms to those of other patients.

Diseases can have two causes: external and internal. Homeopathy emphasizes the internal cause of the disease. It is mostly concerned with the primary functional aspect of the disease, the initial disturbance, the cause, and not just the secondary symptoms, such as the headache. Therefore, in homeopathy, the emphasis is on distinguishing the primary symptoms, which represent the disease process itself, from the secondary symptoms, which are just the outward manifestation of what is taking place inside the body. In fact, symptoms are not seen as being caused by the disease, but are seen as expressions of the curative powers of the individual in an attempt to heal his or her body.

If you have hay fever, which is a secondary symptom, the homeopathic approach will be to assess what led to the disruption of the vital energy within your body, since that is what caused the development of the runny nose and the other symptoms. Instead of taking medications to reduce or suppress the symptoms, the homeopathic approach is to view the symptoms as indicative of the deranged internal environment of health. Similarly, in a patient suffering from headache, the homeopathic approach determines the functional symptoms (primary disease) that have led to the secondary symptom (the headache). Classic homeopathy addresses the totality of the functional symptoms of the disease and uses the symptoms as the basis of curative treatment. For the homeopathic physician, the objective is to decipher the true symptoms of the patient, not the outward manifestation of the true symptoms.

In homeopathy, the symptoms are classified into three types: common, general, and particular:

1. **Common** symptoms are the symptoms that bring you to the doctor's office, such as headache or fever, but these symptoms are the least important when selecting a remedy.

2. In contrast, **general** symptoms are the ones that a homeopathic physician is most concerned with. These symptoms describe your overall feeling of illness or wellbeing. Mental symptoms are very important, as your mental state is a strong reflection of how healthy or unwell your body is. The most important symptoms are the general symptoms that pertain to the individual as a whole. The degree of success that a physician will have in determining proper treatment is based on skill and patience in uncovering the total symptom picture.

3. The **particular** symptoms are those that pertain to a specific organ, but they are not as significant as the general symptoms in choosing a remedy. The homeopathic physician looks for any strange or peculiar symptoms that set you apart from other patients with similar symptoms.

The sequence of the symptoms is critical, and, especially in chronic cases, the initial symptoms that preceded the current state are of utmost importance. For example, if a patient is suffering from headaches, the homeopathic physician is not just concerned with the current symptoms; he or she needs to know when the headaches first began, and what may have led to the headaches. The remedy will be based on the initial symptoms rather than the current symptomatology. The treatment is not based on one symptom alone, but on the totality of the symptom picture. In diagnosing the patient, the objective is not to fit the symptoms into a specific disease and then treat the disease, but to use the totality of the symptoms to figure out the characteristics and personality of the patient.

Homeopathy is based on the following fundamental laws:

1. **The first law** is that *like cures like*, or more accurately, *let like be cured by like*. According to this law, the primary symptoms of the diseases are cured by a drug that produces the same symptoms in a healthy human being.
2. **The second law** is that cure takes place in a particular order: from an important organ to a less important organ, and symptoms disappear in the reverse order of their appearance, the first to appear being the last to disappear.
3. **The third law** is that the quantity of action necessary to affect a change in nature is the one that has the least impact. Very minute quantities can affect profound change. As a corollary, the quantity of drug required is in inverse ratio to the similarity of the patient's symptoms to the symptoms caused by that drug in a healthy individual. The greater the similarity of the symptoms the drug produces in a healthy individual to those of the patient, the lesser the quantity of the drug required.
4. **The fourth law** is that functional symptoms always precede structural symptoms. Here the functional symptoms are those that are related to the internal organ affected by the illness or disease.

Homeopathic Treatment

Homeopathy is very physician-dependent. The skilled homeopathic physician has to be a good listener and a master at cross-examination as well as a good observer, carefully noting every movement and expression of the patient.

Homeopathic medications are based on the principle that the proper dose of a drug is the minimum amount that will stimulate the body's vital energy to react against the disease and bring about a state of health. In practical terms, it is the minimum dose required to produce a slight aggravation of the symptoms. In order to get to the minimum dose, the medications are diluted many times. This process of successive dilutions is called *potentization*. The higher the potency, the lower the concentration of the original medicine.

Homeopathic remedies are found in several forms:

1. *Mother tinctures*, which are alcohol extracts of the original substance
2. *Triturations*, which are ground-up powders of the original substance, or tablets made of powder
3. *Tablets* (or pillules), which are sugar tablets on which a few drops of the liquid form of the potentized remedy are placed
4. *Globules*, which are larger sugar tablets prepared similarly to the tablets

After selecting the appropriate remedy, the next task is to select the proper potency and administer it in the form most suitable for the patient. Only one single dose of the remedy is given, after which the homeopath waits for a response. In acute diseases, the reaction can occur within a few minutes.

There are some substances that you should avoid when taking homeopathic remedies. Certain substances with strong odors, such as coffee, strong smelling herbs, teas, nicotine, and excessive alcohol can interfere with the homeopathic remedy. There should be a proper time gap between taking these types of substances and the homeopathic remedy. In addition, you should rinse your mouth before taking the remedy to clear your mouth of any food particle or odor.

We have purposefully avoided discussing specific homeopathic remedies because all homeopathic treatment is directed toward each individual patient and his or her unique characteristics. What has caused the disturbance in your internal homeostasis is unique to you. However, in most cases, the cause of the disturbance can be traced to poor living habits: poor diet, lack of exercise, excessive stress, exposure to toxins, whether inhaled, consumed, or any other kind of exposure, and other aspects of your lifestyle that have affected your spirit and your mind. Homeopathic remedies can help to restore the balance, but you need to facilitate the treatment by improving your daily living habits, and thus your lifestyle.

In our practice, many patients have responded so favorably to homeopathic remedies that they have been able to stop or greatly reduce their dependence on medications.

Section IV

SPECIAL SITUATIONS

CHAPTER 27

Headache in Women

- The greatest barrier to effective management is under-recognition; headaches may be thought of as a natural part of a woman's menstrual cycle or *premenstrual syndrome* (PMS), or it may be due to *lack of patient awareness* about migraines related to menstruation.
- Patients with menstrual migraine are at greatest risk for headache during the two days prior to onset of menstruation and three days following the onset.
- Some of the non-pharmacologic measures that have proven effective in managing headaches in pregnancy include avoiding sudden movements, maintaining blood glucose levels, breathing fresh air, relaxation and massage, acupuncture, homeopathy, stress management, and lifestyle modification.

H eadache is very common in women. Approximately 70 percent of migraine sufferers are female. As we have discussed, migraine patients are sensitive to external and internal triggers. Hormones play an important role in these types of headaches. Different hormonal changes occur at different stages of a woman's life. Each of these stages—menarche and the menstrual cycle, pregnancy, perimenopause and postmenopause—has associated headache events. It is presumed that the changes in hormonal levels are responsible for triggering many of the headaches suffered by women.

Sudden changes in estrogen levels are not good for migraine headaches. Studies have shown that a drop in estrogen levels triggers the migraine headache in most women. The actual level of estrogen, whether high or low, is not as important as the dramatic changes in the levels, either up or down.

Menstrual Migraine

Menstrual migraine is a specific condition unique to women. Although it is not a separate category under the classification of the International Headache Society (IHS), the IHS does recognize that "migraine without aura may occur almost exclusively at a particular time of the menstrual cycle—so-called menstrual migraine." Let us now examine what is unique about menstrual migraine.

There are two types of migraines associated with menstruation: pure menstrual migraine and menstrually related migraine. Both of these are migraine without aura. By definition, *pure menstrual migraine* is migraine which occurs exclusively during the five-to-six-day perimenstrual period (within fewer than two days before the onset of menses and up to four or five days after the onset of menses) and at no other time. This type of migraine is rare. *Menstrually related migraine* is defined as migraine occurring during both the perimenstrual period and at other times of the month. However, the management and treatment of both are similar, and unless otherwise noted, we will be referring to them collectively as *menstrual migraine.*

Among female migraneurs, approximately 60 percent of headaches are menstrual migraine, and only 40 percent are non-menstrual. As mentioned in the chapter on epidemiology, following puberty, migraine affects 27 percent of women and 9 percent of men. The hormone fluctuations that trigger migraine at puberty are also associated with a greater incidence of migraine at the time of menstruation. The majority of women who suffer from recurrent migraine have increased risk of headaches at the time of their menses. Sometimes, though, these menstrual migraines are not recognized, and as a result may not be treated. Menstrual migraines tend to be more severe, last longer, and are more difficult to treat.

Most women who suffer menstrual migraine have migraine-associated disability, causing significant limitations in their daily activities. In addition, migraine attacks occurring at the time of menstruation are more severe in their intensity and duration, and have a greater resistance to treatment.

Barrier to Effective Management

By far, the greatest barrier to effective management is under-recognition, as both patients and physicians may mistakenly diagnose menstrual headaches as a natural part of their menstrual cycle or *premenstrual syndrome* (PMS). Another important reason for this under-recognition is *lack of patient awareness* about menstrual migraine.

The mechanisms causing menstrual migraine are not entirely understood. It is thought that the rapid fluctuations in the levels of estrogen and progesterone cause the headache, specifically, the rapidly declining levels of estrogen that occur prior to the menstrual period. The brain's response to the declining levels of estrogen is the trigger for the headache, not the reduced level of estrogen. These hormones signal the uterus to increase production of prostaglandins, which are thought to be responsible for the pain. The hormone fluctuations also trigger a cascade of responses in the brain, which include impaired metabolism of different neurotransmitters (serotonin, dopamine, opioid, and melatonin to name a few).

If you are a woman suffering from severe headaches, the most accurate way of determining whether you have menstrual migraine is to keep a headache diary. Track your menstrual cycle and other possible headache triggers, and notate the days you have a headache. Some women do not remember the exact dates of their menstrual cycle, so a calendar is very helpful in correlating the headache with the menstrual cycle. This diary is very helpful in devising an appropriate treatment plan.

Birth control pills (BCP) and hormone replacement therapy (HRT), especially those containing high doses of estrogen, can be important headache triggers in many women. Some women who do not suffer generally from headaches may actually start experiencing a headache for the first time after starting BCPs. The headache characteristics may also change with the use of BCPs.

Treatment of Menstrual Migraine

For the acute treatment of menstrual migraine, the recommendations are the same as for other types of migraine. The goal of acute therapy is to stop the headache before it becomes a headache. Mefanamic acid, at a dose of 800 milligrams every eight hours, was found in one study to be very effective. Approximately 80 percent of patients with menstrual migraine experienced relief of the headache at two hours compared to only 17 percent response with placebo. Early treatment with triptans in the evolution of the headache offers greater pain relief than treatment given after the migraine pain has started. Almost all the triptans, but especially sumatriptan, zolmitriptan, and rizatriptan, have been shown to have good efficacy in menstrual migraine. A short-acting triptan can be followed a few hours later with a longer-acting triptan (such as frovatriptan). DHE has also been found to have similar effectiveness as the triptans.

Short-Term Prevention

Women with menstrual migraine are at greatest risk for headache during the two days prior to the onset of menstruation and three days following the onset. Short-term prevention therapy provides protection during the days patients are at greatest risk of headache. Keep in mind that there are no medications approved for this type of indication by the FDA.

Medications that have been studied for this type of short-term prevention include naratriptan, sumatriptan, and frovatriptan. The guidelines for the use of triptans state that triptans should not be taken for more than two days per week. However, this does not mean that other triptans or other medications like **NSAIDs** are not useful. This is one of the cases where taking a triptan for a few days is appropriate and generally will not lead to a medication overuse headache. Naproxen and magnesium have also been proven effective for short-term prevention. For patients who have low magnesium, supplemental magnesium given fifteen days prior to menstruation has also been shown to reduce the number of days with headache. In addition to medications, it is important to avoid migraine triggers, such as sleep deprivation, dehydration, and hunger, among others.

The most effective therapy, however, is to treat the monthly fluctuations of estrogen. HRT with an estrogen supplement can smooth out the levels of estrogen. Sometimes, taking a BCP for regulating your menstrual cycle can reduce your headaches. However, if you suffer from migraine with aura, keep in mind that BCP increases the risk of stroke. Extended-cycle dosing of combined hormonal contraceptives has been proven effective as a preventative strategy. Combining this with estrogen supplementation during menstrual drop in levels has also been effective.

A particularly useful treatment for menstrual headache is supplementation with Vitamin E. This vitamin stabilizes estrogen levels and can help prevent menstrual migraines. Taking high doses of the vitamin around the time of menstruation, such as 800 international units (IUs), can be very effective.

Carefully chosen hormone therapy, such as a combination of bio-identical estrogen with a bio-identical progestin, can bring significant relief from menstrual migraine. Since the headache occurs due to a drop in estrogen level, supplementing the estrogen at the right time is crucial. Scientific data has been conflicting as to the efficacy of estrogen therapy. It has been suggested that the dose of estrogen in most studies was too low to show good efficacy; there is some evidence that using Estradiol 0.1 mg instead of 0.05 mg is more effective in reducing headaches. The form of estrogen delivery can make a difference as well. The estrogen patch seems to provide a more consistent blood level of estrogen than the other forms—the capsule, pill, or ring. Estradiol gel 1.5 mg applied daily for short-term prophylaxis, starting at two to three days prior to menstruation for a total of seven days has shown in experimental studies to be effective in preventing headaches. There is also some evidence that synthetic hormones may not work as effectively as bio-identical hormones.

According to conventional medicine, the best therapeutic strategy for treatment of menstrual migraine is to first treat with acute, abortive therapies to stop the headache and employ short-term prevention when abortive treatment is not sufficient to control the symptoms. Long-term prevention should be initiated only if short-term prevention is not effective.

In women who are unable to predict their menstrual cycle, continuous prophylaxis using Estradiol implants has been very effective in maintaining stable, high estrogen levels, thereby decreasing menstrual migraines.

Headaches During pregnancy

Headaches are common during pregnancy. Changes in hormone levels can cause new headaches in a patient who has never had headaches before. However, in approximately 50 percent of women with migraine headaches, the headaches actually improve during pregnancy, especially in the second and third trimesters. This is thought to be due to the lack of fluctuation in the estrogen levels during pregnancy. Estrogen acts as a pain modulator, decreasing pain perception. Some women, though, do experience worsening of the headache frequency and/or intensity during pregnancy. The headaches in pregnancy can occur suddenly, without any warning, and stop just as suddenly. They can be tension-type headaches or migraines. The duration can also vary from minutes to hours to days. In short, you can have any type of headache during pregnancy; furthermore, it is often hard to predict who will have them, and what the frequency, intensity, and duration will be.

Causes of Headaches During Pregnancy

Patients who suffer from migraine headaches already have a lowered threshold and increased sensitivity to triggers, both internal and external. Estrogen influences other organ systems, which may increase headache susceptibility. Estrogen increases the susceptibility of the blood vessels to constrict. However, there are other causes as well. There are many associated emotional and physical changes during pregnancy, and these can contribute to the increased frequency of tension-type headaches. Patients who have a history of migraine headaches, but whose headaches had been well controlled with preventative medications prior to pregnancy, may notice an exacerbation of their headaches after stopping their medications during pregnancy.

Most of the headaches that occur during the first two trimesters are generally not severe and do not require any specific treatment. If women are still suffering from headaches at the end of the first trimester, they will likely not improve substantially during the remainder of the pregnancy. Headaches occurring primarily during the third trimester can be more serious due to underlying high blood pressure, especially if they are severe, persistent, and accompanied by blurred vision.

Post-Partum Headaches

More than half of post-partum headaches are the typical headaches the patient was suffering from before pregnancy. But there are some serious causes that need to be considered that can be life-threatening, especially if there are focal neurological deficits. More women are getting epidural injections for their delivery, and this can lead to an increased risk of low-pressure headache.

In the post-partum period, the hormonal changes begin again, and the patient's susceptibility to the hormonal changes reverts to her body's pre-pregnancy state. Headaches may be frequent during the first week postpartum. These headaches are most likely related to the rapid decrease in estrogen following delivery. Some women with headaches also become depressed in the immediate postpartum period.

The most important secondary cause of post-partum headaches is pre-eclampsia/eclampsia, although the headache is usually not the first symptom of this condition. Other serious causes, such as venous sinus thrombosis, pituitary apoplexy, or subarachnoid hemorrhage, or the newly recognized condition known as reversible cerebral vasoconstriction syndrome, should also be considered. If you start having significant headaches in the post-partum period, it is critical to see a physician so that these potentially life-threatening causes can be ruled out.

Treatment Strategies

Most of the headaches occurring during pregnancy do not require any drug treatment. Most women are reluctant to taking medications during pregnancy anyway, due to the possible teratogenic (bringing harm to the growing fetus) side effects of the medications. Fortunately, the majority of the headaches can be managed by non-pharmacologic strategies.

Some of the measures that can be helpful in managing headaches are the following:

1. **Avoiding sudden movements:** Any movement that decreases the blood flow to the brain, such as suddenly standing from a sitting position, can cause headaches and other symptoms such as dizziness. In normal conditions (when not pregnant), standing up suddenly triggers a compensatory mechanism in the body that maintains adequate blood flow to the brain. However, in pregnancy, the uterus gets preferential treatment. When blood pressure suddenly drops upon standing up, the blood flow to the uterus gets preference over the brain. So, you may suddenly feel faint, become dizzy, and get a headache when you get up suddenly from a sitting position. In order to minimize these symptoms, it is important that you move slowly when getting up.

2. **Maintaining blood glucose levels:** As we discussed in the chapter on diet, hunger can cause headaches. During pregnancy, the tendency to develop low blood sugar (hypoglycemia) is increased, which means there is a higher chance of developing headaches. One way to maintain adequate blood glucose levels is to consume carbohydrates with a low glycemic index so that hypoglycemia can be minimized.

3. **Breathing fresh air:** Poorly ventilated, overheated, smoke-filled rooms can cause sinus congestion and resultant headaches. Get out of the house or office and breathe in plenty of fresh air.

4. **Relaxation and massage:** Getting a head massage can be very therapeutic. Different relaxation strategies have been found to be particularly useful in successfully treating headaches. This issue has been

adequately covered in the chapter on relaxation. Biofeedback has also been utilized for this purpose.

5. **Acupuncture:** As discussed in the chapter on acupuncture, this is a very safe treatment during pregnancy. It is actually used to balance the energy fluctuations that occur during pregnancy, and can be safely used for treatment of headaches that do not resolve with other general measures.

6. **Homeopathy:** This is also a safe treatment for pregnant women. The homeopathic remedies are diluted so much that there is practically no danger to the mother or the fetus.

7. **Stress management:** Stress is the number-one trigger for both tension-type and migraine headaches. Stress management can be helpful in controlling the negative side of stress and in helping you focus more on the positive. We recommend that you read the chapter on stress management to learn appropriate stress-relieving strategies.

8. **Lifestyle modification:** To minimize headaches during pregnancy, eat a well-balanced, low-fat, low-sugar diet; avoid skipping meals; avoid alcohol, caffeine, and nicotine; and get adequate sleep and exercise. Overly restrictive diets or elimination diets can have a negative effect on the growing fetus, so care should be taken in maintaining adequate, proper nutrition.

Although medications should be avoided during pregnancy, sometimes the non-pharmacologic measures may not be effective in controlling your headaches. If medications have to be taken, you should avoid taking them too regularly.

Safe Medications During Pregnancy

Medications are assigned a pregnancy risk category of either A, B, C, D, or X. Category A drugs are the least risky and have been shown in human studies to be safe. The safest medications during pregnancy are acetaminophen (Tylenol), short-acting opioids (such as Tylenol with codeine), and anti-nausea medications. The other common medications such as NSAIDs and aspirin should not be taken during pregnancy because of their tendency to cause bleeding or uterine contractions. Triptans have not been studied extensively in pregnancy; however, patients who have taken them have not reported any adverse effects of the medications to the fetus (as of the time of this writing). Because of lack of long-term safety data, though, they have been designated as category C. According to current thought, sporadic use of sumatriptan is a safe option. After the first trimester, most of the NSAIDs, butorphanol, and narcotics are relatively safe.

Of the preventative medications, beta-blockers (such as propranolol) have been used widely during pregnancy without any untoward effects. Unfortunately, there are no category A preventative medications. These drugs are also used to treat blood pressure during pregnancy. Some medications such as valproate are contraindicated during pregnancy because of their high risk for causing serious side effects. There is insufficient evidence to recommend other preventative medications such as antidepressants and anti-seizure medications. The risk of taking medications belonging to categories C, D, and X is high. Category C medications have shown some problems in animal studies, but no problems in humans so far. Categories D and X should be avoided in pregnancy because of suspected or known risks to the developing fetus.

Having said all that, there are instances where exceptions have to be made. Eventually, the best course of action is to take medications that have the least risk associated with them and use the lowest dose that provides headache relief. You need to be treated by an experienced headache specialist who can monitor your health and find the best possible treatment.

In these instances, non-pharmacologic treatments may be particularly helpful, especially acupuncture, as it not only helps the headache, but also regulates the energy disturbances that result from pregnancy in the absence of a headache. It can be considered an acute treatment and a preventative, as it can treat the energy fluctuations before they have a chance to trigger the headache. Homeopathy also belongs to this category of safe alternatives during pregnancy.

Menopause

As women approach menopause, the estrogen fluctuations gradually decrease, resulting in decreased frequency of headaches. Headaches may resolve with menopause. In fact, anywhere from 30 to 70 percent of women can experience a dramatic decrease in the frequency of their headaches, and some achieve headache freedom. However, during the period just before menopause, known as the perimenopause, headaches can increase significantly. Perimenopause is a tough period for most women. This is when most of the problems associated with menopause are most prominent: mood changes, hot flashes, depression, and the like. This is also the time when patients can start having medication overuse headaches (MOH). Some women may experience the opposite, although that is not as common. In women who receive hormone replacement therapy (HRT), the headaches may not improve with menopause, as the body's estrogen is replaced by the HRT. Patients may in fact notice an initial increase in the headache frequency upon starting HRT. Because of the other possible side effects of HRT, we recommend that patients check with their headache specialist before taking HRT, and to use the lowest possible dose of estrogen on a daily basis to reduce the fluctuations.

CHAPTER 28
Headaches in Children and Adolescents

- Children younger than three years usually experience secondary headache, which means there is probably an underlying cause that needs to be examined by a professional.
- The most common cause of acute recurrent headache is migraine with or without aura.
- Migraine headache usually begins in childhood. Besides pharmacologic treatments, reassuring the patient's family of the benign nature of the headache is of utmost importance.
- Alternative treatments including acupuncture, NAET, and homeopathy are particularly effective in treating children.

K ids get headaches too! If you are the parent of a child with headaches, you know how true that statement is. As a parent, you might be struggling with whether the child is suffering from just a simple headache or a more ominous underlying medical problem. We hope this chapter clarifies some issues and gives you some answers before you get too concerned.

Childhood headaches are common, and they increase in adolescence. Approximately one third of children who are at least seven years of age and 50 percent of those who are at least fifteen years of age have headaches. In a recent study, the prevalence of headache was found to be in the range of 37 percent to 51 percent in children who were at least seven years of age, which gradually rose to 57 percent to 82 percent by age fifteen. Before puberty, boys are affected more frequently than girls are, but after the onset of puberty, headaches occur more frequently in girls. Fortunately, the majority of the childhood headaches resolve quickly. In some children, they may be severe enough to require medical evaluation.

Approximately 75 percent of children's headaches are TTH, and only 25 percent are migraine. Children with migraine are usually pale, quiet, or grouchy, complaining of light and sound sensitivity, and may have nausea, vomiting, and loss of appetite. Similar to adults, they want to lie down in a dark, quiet area. However, attacks of migraine in childhood differ in location and duration from adult patients. Children frequently have pain on both sides (bilateral), and mainly in the forehead region, and the duration is shorter. Other associated symptoms in children include abdominal pain, anorexia, pallor, and a desire to sleep. Typical triggers include school-related stress, lack of sleep, minor head trauma, anxiety, fatigue, and a whole host of other triggers common to adults. Children may be more sensitive to car or motion sickness, and if they have a family history of migraines, may develop migraine headaches later.

Medical research has described five distinct temporal patterns of headache in children. These are:

1. **Acute headache**: This is a single episode of headache without any previous history of headaches.
2. **Acute recurrent headache**: This represents repeated episodes of headache with normal, headache-free intervening periods.
3. **Chronic progressive headache**: This type of headache steadily worsens in severity and frequency over time.

4. **Chronic daily headaches**: This represents frequent headaches or constant headache without any significant relief.
5. **Mixed headache**: This type consists of migraine-type headaches superimposed on a background of low-grade, constant TTH.

There are certain presentations of migraine that are unique to children. Some children may experience repeated attacks of intense nausea and vomiting, which may be associated with tiredness and fatigue. These headaches are similar from attack to attack. The characteristic feature that sets them apart from other conditions causing nausea and vomiting is that there is complete resolution of symptoms between attacks. This is known as *cyclic vomiting syndrome*, and is a childhood precursor for migraine headaches.

Another unique presentation of migraine in children is a condition called *abdominal migraine*. This is a condition where children experience repeated attacks of severe abdominal pain associated with nausea and vomiting without any associated headache. The child is completely normal when the abdominal pain resolves.

Laboratory tests, including EEG, CT scans, MRI, and lumbar puncture, can be done as needed to evaluate the reason for your child's headaches. The appropriate test will be obtained after a thorough evaluation.

Psychological evaluation may be helpful in children and adolescents suffering from chronic daily headaches and mixed-headache patterns to assess for possible stress-related situations and to determine if psychological counseling or other related therapies would be of any benefit.

Children younger than three years usually have secondary headaches, meaning there is an underlying cause that needs to be examined by a medical professional. Children with acute evolution of headache accompanied by focal neurologic symptoms or signs (morning vomiting, headaches that awaken the child) should also be referred to a specialist in headache management. Children or adolescents with chronic-progressive headaches, where the headache worsens over time without any improvement and can be associated with increasing intracranial pressure, also should be referred to a specialist.

Treatment

Fortunately, most headaches in children are not due to any serious underlying problem, and are easily managed. For acute recurrent headache, the treatment is directed at symptomatic relief of the pain. The most common cause of acute recurrent headache is migraine with or without aura. Migraine headache usually begins in childhood. Besides pharmacologic treatments, reassuring the patient's family of the benign nature of the headache is of utmost importance. As with any other migraine patient, identifying the possible triggers and limiting exposure to those triggers is important. The triggers in children can be disrupted sleep, stress, and skipping meals. Getting adequate sleep is very beneficial and may obviate the need for medications. Dietary triggers can be difficult to avoid, as young patients may not understand elimination diets. It is important to limit the child's consumption of caffeine and sugar. In these cases, treatment with acupuncture and NAET can be exceptionally helpful.

If the headache does not resolve with non-pharmacologic measures, treatment with medications may be necessary. Generally, we tend to avoid medicating children, as they can be exceptionally sensitive to side effects. If children need to be treated with drugs, analgesics such as acetaminophen (Tylenol), ibuprofen (Advil, Motrin), or triptans can be used sparingly. Not all of the triptans have been approved by FDA for use in children, but they have shown to be safe medications, and can be quite effective. Rizatriptan is approved for use in children, and almotriptan is approved for use in both children and adolescents.

In a minority of children, the headaches are frequent and non-responsive to general measures or acute medications. In these cases, preventative therapy may need to be considered. The same drugs used for prevention in adults, such as topiramate, valproate, and beta-blockers, can be used in children. Of course, the dosages need to be modified for children. Amitriptyline (brand name Elavil) or propranolol are recommended over other drugs for preventing headaches in children. Valproate is used less frequently because it has slightly more side effects in children. Cyproheptadine (brand name Periactin) has also been used as a preventative agent. We cannot overemphasize the benefit of using alternative therapies such as acupuncture, homeopathy, and NAET in these situations. They can be highly efficacious and safe alternatives to drug treatments. In addition, stress management strategies, including biofeedback, have been used successfully in children. Improving the quality of sleep and regular exercise are also important factors that will help in treating the headaches and related conditions.

Cluster headaches are rare in children and adolescents.

For **chronic progressive headaches**, the approach to treatment can be different. Since the headaches are steadily increasing in intensity and frequency, it is critical to perform an imaging study to assess for a possible underlying brain abnormality. The treatment and management depend on the results of the imaging study. The cause of these headaches can range from overuse of medications to brain tumor.

For **chronic daily headache**, the treatment can be particularly challenging. It is especially important to assess for any underlying psychological reason. Children should undergo a detailed evaluation of sleep patterns, dietary habits, stress-producing factors, exercise habits, and societal interactions, as well as testing for illicit drug use.

In cyclic vomiting syndrome and abdominal migraine, the focus is on aggressive hydration and the use of anti-emetic agents to counter the nausea and vomiting. Triptans can be effective although no triptan has been approved for these two variants of migraine headaches.

CHAPTER 29
Chronic Daily Headaches

- The symptoms that accompany chronic migraine include gastrointestinal complaints, aches and pains in various muscles and bones, and psychological symptoms such as depression.
- Medications employed for the treatment of CDH belong to the category of preventative medications, which include antiepileptic drugs, antidepressants, and opioids.
- CDH is an ideal state for exploring alternative strategies, as in most cases, the drugs themselves are part of the problem.
- Best response is achieved through an intensive program that includes acupuncture, NAET, herbal supplements, chiropractic treatment, mind-body exercises including yoga and meditation, and lifestyle changes including nutrition and homeopathy.

People who come to a specialized headache clinic are usually referred because their headaches are not controllable through standard approaches. A majority of these people have mixed headaches, or coexistent migraine and tension-type headaches. It is estimated that approximately 4 to 5 percent of adults suffer from Chronic Daily Headaches (CDH).

CDH are defined as headaches lasting at least four hours on fifteen or more days out of the month. However, as the name suggests, most people with CDH suffer from chronic daily headaches, which are present twenty-four hours a day, seven days a week. These people have generally been difficult to treat, and are an endless cause of frustration for themselves and their treating physicians. They are a bane of emergency room physicians, as they end up there repeatedly because of lack of response to standard medications. No specific therapies have been approved by the FDA for treatment of CDH. Most of the medications used for their treatment are used off-label (drugs that are used for a condition for which they have not been approved). Let us first examine who is at risk for developing CDH before we discuss specific treatment strategies.

Chronic daily headaches are more common in women, especially those of Caucasian descent. The most significant risk factor is obesity and a previous history of frequent headaches. People who have suffered minor head trauma also seem to be at a higher risk of developing CDH. There is also an association with psychiatric disorders, such as depression and anxiety. CDH are also associated with major life changes, such as moving and divorce, as well as sleep changes, smoking, and increased caffeine intake.

CDH does not fit into the classic definitions of either TTH or migraine. In fact, CDH can be of different types including chronic migraine, chronic tension-type (CTTH), chronic posttraumatic headache, and cluster headache. Many people with CDH may be suffering from medication overuse headache.

Secondary Causes of CDH

It goes without saying that when people develop CDH, we need to consider a possible underlying cause or etiology. Some secondary causes can mimic CDH. The possibilities given in Table 1 need to be considered.

Causes of Secondary CDH

1. Post-traumatic (after head trauma)
2. Cervical spine disease with radiculopathy (pinched nerve in the neck)
3. TMJ syndrome
4. Inflammation of the temporal arteries (temporal arteritis)
5. Brain hemorrhage
6. Brain tumor
7. Infections in the brain
8. Vascular malformations
9. Intracranial high blood pressure
10. Intracranial low blood pressure

All of these conditions can be confounded by medication overuse.

Symptoms of CDH

When migraine patients develop chronic migraine, they may notice some new symptoms in addition to the ones commonly experienced as part of the headache syndrome. The symptoms that accompany chronic migraine include gastrointestinal complaints, aches and pains in various muscles and bones, and psychological symptoms such as depression. These people usually become dependent on medication, sometimes taking combination drugs containing acetaminophen, aspirin, and caffeine many times daily. They frequently require treatment for dependence on these drugs in addition to treatment for their headaches. With any type of CDH, the headache is usually present in the morning upon awakening and stays throughout the day. Migraine patients usually have migraine without aura.

New Daily Persistent Headache

New Daily Persistent Headache (NDPH) is a subtype of CDH. It begins suddenly one day and does not remit. It is persistent and usually refractory to treatment. It is more common in women. It affects women in their twenties and thirties. When it affects men, it tends to be later in life, in their fifties. The characteristics of the pain are variable. It can have features of both TTH and migraine. People who suffer from this remember exactly when the headaches began. There is no prior history of headaches and no known underlying cause. Fortunately, it is very rare.

Table 1: Features of Chronic Migraine and CTTH

Feature	Chronic Migraine	Chronic Tension-type Headache
Location	Unilateral	Bilateral
Pain characteristics	Throbbing	Tightening, pressure-type pain
Nausea and/or vomiting	Present	Only mild nausea (if at all)
Sensitivity to light	Usually present	May be present
Sensitivity to sound	Usually present	May be present
Severity	Moderate-severe	Mild to moderate
Aggravated by routine physical activity	Yes	No
Anxiety and/or depression	Yes	Possibly
Sleep disturbance	Very common	Less common
Musculoskeletal symptoms	Yes	Less common

Hemicrania Continua

In the classification of CDH, there is another type of headache worth mentioning called Hemicrania Continua. It is described as pain on one side of the head that can be particularly severe. The severity can fluctuate from mild to severe. As the name suggests, it occurs on only one side of the head, and usually stays on the same side. The pain is continuous without any pain-free periods. Pain exacerbations are usually accompanied by autonomic features, which include runny nose with nasal congestion, tearing (lacrimation), eye redness, eye discomfort, sweating, and drooping eyelids. The pain is similar to migraine, including the associated symptoms of nausea, vomiting, and sensitivity to light and sound.

Treatment of CDH

A multitude of medications are available for treatment of chronic headache, but none of them have been approved by the FDA for this condition. Most headache specialists base their treatment on their own experience since there is no good evidence-based medicine (EBM) for the use of specific drugs. There are currently ongoing clinical trials that may shed light on the most appropriate drug treatments in the near future.

The drug treatment approach is to first establish the diagnosis. Once it has been established, the optimal treatment includes ascertaining concomitant medical problems such as a mood disorder (anxiety, depression), pain elsewhere in the body (neck/back pain, fibromyalgia), sleep disturbances (difficulty falling asleep, waking up early, sleep apnea), as well as assessing medication usage to consider the possibility of medication overuse headache.

Most people with CDH have already become resistant to treatment with both OTC and prescription painkillers. Many of them have been consuming large amounts of non-opioid and opioid analgesics on a daily basis with minimal relief. But stopping the medications causes increased intensity of the pain as their bodies develop tolerance to the medications. People first need to be detoxified from these addictive medications, which can be a formidable task. The treatment can only be effective when the patient forms a partnership with his or her doctor and remains committed to it.

Fortunately, there are effective treatment choices for providing relief from the pain. There is no quick fix. Let us discuss the various strategies, and then we can come up with an individualized plan of treatment for your particular situation.

Drug Treatments for CDH

Medications employed in the treatment of CDH belong to the category of preventative medications. Acute medications are generally avoided, as they might themselves be part of the problem. As discussed earlier, preventative drugs, the medications generally considered for treatment, belong to one of three categories: antiepileptic drugs, antidepressants, and beta-blockers.

Antiepileptic drugs: Divalproate has shown more effectiveness in preventing chronic migraine than CTTH. Studies with topiramate are still undergoing, but it has shown promise in decreasing the pain in CDH. Other antiepileptic drugs, such as lamotrigine (brand name Lamictal) and levetiracetam (brand name Keppra), have also been tried, but so far there is no scientific data except for anecdotal evidence of their use in CDH.

These medications do not show benefit immediately upon taking them, as would be expected from acute medications. They have to be taken daily, sometimes twice daily, depending on the medication, in order to decrease the sensitivity of the brain and reduce the frequency, duration, and intensity of the headaches. It is beneficial in these circumstances to keep a headache diary to chart your progress. All too often, people give up on these medications without giving them an adequate trial.

More recently, combining two different preventative medications has shown to be more effective than single agent therapy. The rationale for using combination therapy is that it can target different underlying mechanisms that cause pain. For example, the combination of a beta-blocker and valproate was shown to be 50 percent more effective in previously resistant patients. In another study, a beta-blocker was combined with topiramate. However, some patients experience more side effects on combination drug therapy.

For chronic migraine patients, onabotulinum toxin A (Botox) has proven to be effective in many cases. It is injected in seven specific head and neck muscles areas through a series of thirty-one injections. The effect generally lasts for up to three months, and then has to be repeated. There are few if any drug interactions.

CDH and Other Alternative Therapies

This is an instance where the best chance of success is in a more comprehensive treatment regimen that includes select alternative strategies, lifestyle management, and stress control. Since drug treatment has been largely unsuccessful, any treatment regimen that does not utilize non-medication strategies will be doomed to failure. In most cases, the drugs themselves have become part of the problem. It is critical to utilize a logical approach to the treatment of this condition. You need to think long-term and root out the cause of headaches. This can be achieved through an intensive program that includes acupuncture, NAET, herbal supplements, chiropractic treatment, mind-body exercises including yoga and meditation, and lifestyle changes including nutritional modification and homeopathy, as these alternatives address the cause more than the symptom. Symptom control is a very small part of the larger problem. If not addressed appropriately, this condition will most likely persist and lead to further deterioration in the patient's vital energy, until a point is reached when the headaches become very hard to treat by any means, and are eventually irreversible. The treatment regimen discussed under our Headache Reduction Program can be very effective in treating CDH.

STRESS AND HEADACHE REDUCTION PROGRAM (SHARP)

CHAPTER 30

The SHARP Approach

Our approach is designed to bring about healing, not just symptom control. However, symptom control is an important aspect of healing. After all, healing cannot occur if you are still suffering from the symptoms of pain.

The SHARP Approach is a healing process that incorporates both acute treatment of the quick fix and lifestyle modification. Before embarking on a life-changing program, you have to stop the acute pain. When you are in agonizing pain, it is difficult even to think. Using an abortive therapy is equally as important as changing your lifestyle to minimize the impact of headaches. A life management program starts with simple steps. Changing habits is not easy; there is an inherent resistance to change. Making drastic changes too quickly seldom leads to long-term results. Therefore, a gradual introduction to lifestyle management while experiencing more rapid symptom control is the preferred method.

As mentioned earlier, disease exists in the physical, mental, emotional, and spiritual realms. Starting the process on a physical level produces the quickest results initially, which is the aforementioned quick fix. However, unless the other three realms are involved in the healing process, the results will be short-lived. An integrative program combines immediate symptom control with long-term lifestyle management. We will not spend time discussing the specifics of symptom control, as most of you are familiar with this approach by now. Symptom control is what the majority of mainstream Western medicine is all about.

There are some general principles that underlie the treatment program. Each of you needs to identify your own personal vulnerabilities and specific lifestyle elements to which you are sensitive. You need to create stability in your lifestyle, as chaos tends to heighten the problem. Stick to a sleep schedule and eat meals at specific times. Any type of disruption to the schedule needs to be anticipated and prepared for.

The time to create patterns of behavior is when you are not suffering from the severe pain of the headache. However, when you are not in pain, the last thing you want to think about is your pain. SHARP gives you practical suggestions that you can gradually incorporate into your lifestyle.

This is an opportunity to examine your life and create harmony between the physical, mental, emotional, and spiritual realms. The headache can be a blessing in disguise as it forces you to create a sense of balance in your life. It forces you to analyze your behavior, your activities, your relationships—in short, your entire existence, to identify factors that lead to your headache. Lifestyle modification involves examining your life and modifying it in a way that eliminates activities that are meaningless while maximizing activities that bring about a sense of satisfaction and meaning to your life.

CHAPTER 31
Lifestyle Management

Headaches are a very complex problem linked closely to a person's lifestyle. They are a symptom of breakdown in our internal milieu, and the most common cause of this is a combination of poor diet, stress, and other facets of unhealthy living. Thus, our approach to treatment of headache starts with lifestyle modification. This approach has proven to be very effective in not only preventing but also curing many conditions, and has the greatest impact on reducing your migraines in the long-term. The dictionary definition of lifestyle is *a manner of living that reflects the attitudes and values of a person or group*. We are dealing here with your attitudes and values as they relate to your health.

Let us focus on how lifestyle modification can help with your headache. Your lifestyle includes your activities of daily living such as eating, sleeping, working, and socializing. In order to make the necessary adjustments, you first need to take stock of what you eat, how you sleep, and how you approach your work and your play.

Diet

What you eat:

Do you live to eat or eat to live? Yes, this may be a philosophical question, but it is not so philosophical when your diet causes physical problems. As noted earlier, what you eat can be either headache promoting or headache preventing. Make sure you understand the differences between the saatvik, tamasic, and rajasic diets. The question is not whether you can eat foods such as chocolate, or drink wine. It is about discovering the foods that are health promoting for you.

Start by first making a critical decision about what types of foods you are going to incorporate into your life, and what types you are going to give up. It will be much more beneficial for you to adopt a saatvik diet. It may take time for your taste buds to accept the change from ice cream to fruits. But without a firm commitment, you may fail in your resolve, as old habits are hard to break.

1. Start following the nine principles of the Headache Prevention Diet as discussed in Chapter 24.
2. What you do while eating food has a big impact on what the food does inside your body.
3. Don't eat to a full stomach. It takes a few minutes for the stomach to send the signal back to the brain to let it know that it is full. If you eat until your hunger is completely gone, you have actually overeaten.
4. Do not shop for food on an empty stomach. You may end up buying more than you require and selecting unhealthy snack foods.

Exercise

We have already seen how exercise lowers the incidence of headache. The increase in oxygenation and glucose uptake by the brain directly affects the neurotransmitters and endorphins that enhance the functioning of the brain. Again, the first step is to decide to exercise. The next step is to get started. It does not really matter what type of exercise you do, as long as you do it regularly. Obviously, the results you get will be in direct proportion to the amount and type of exercise you do; however, doing any type of exercise is better than doing nothing at all.

The first step is to gauge your fitness level and design a program that is appropriate for you. If you have not exercised for some time, you may need to see your physician before you begin any physical fitness program. This is true especially if you suffer from heart disease, dizziness, high blood pressure, a bone or joint problem that could be aggravated by exercise, or if you are over the age of forty and have not exercised in recent years.

As mentioned earlier, there are three aspects of physical fitness: flexibility, strength, and stamina. **Flexibility**, defined as the range of motion of a joint, allows you to perform physical activities with ease. Any exercise program should include exercises that promote flexibility to keep your joints healthy. **Strength** is the ability of a muscle to perform the same action repeatedly. The most important muscles that provide the foundation for all other types of exercise are the muscles of the stomach, trunk, and the shoulders. **Stamina** is defined as the capability of sustaining prolonged stressful effort. It is a measure of how efficient your heart and lungs are in transporting oxygen to your muscles and organs. It is manifested in your overall energy level as well as in your ability to sustain vigorous exercise.

Your exercise program should contain elements that enhance all three aspects: flexibility, strength, and stamina. Flexibility is the foundation of health, in that it lengthens muscles that have contracted due to tension, stress, aging, or injury, while strength does the opposite: it shortens muscles that have been lengthened due to disuse or injury. Working on both provides a balance in the body. Stamina is important for your cardiovascular health; an unconditioned heart has to work harder to do the same amount of work.

An exercise program should make you feel good and reduce your stress, anxiety, and tension. Any headache reduction program will contain exercises that provide a balance of activities to develop your flexibility, strength, and stamina. Plan to work out at least every other day. SHARP provides a personalized exercise program that incorporates proper breathing, yoga, and physical exercise in a balanced manner that develops your flexibility, strength, and stamina. It is beyond the scope of this book to provide you with a detailed exercise program designed for you. However, the information provided should enable you to find a program best suited for you.

Sleep

The human body cannot function without adequate sleep. It is a mandatory period of becoming unconscious to the outer world. Although what really happens while we are asleep is not understood fully, when we do not get enough sleep, several bodily functions begin to deteriorate. Missing one or a few days of adequate sleep is not going to kill you; however, it can severely limit optimal functioning of the brain. You may have experienced the effects of lack of sleep yourself. One thing is certain: your body can become more prone to diseases if you do not get enough sleep. Headache is a common result of sleep deprivation. Getting an adequate amount of sleep is important in controlling all different types of headaches.

Insomnia is a big problem in our society. If you cannot get a good night's sleep, you are not alone. According to the National Institutes of Health, nearly twenty million people in the United States suffer some form of insomnia! However, taking sleeping pills is not always the answer. It is important to first talk to your physician to determine if you may have an underlying sleep disorder that requires medical treatment.

For headache sufferers, good sleep hygiene is a critical element of lifestyle modification. It is not enough to get only the right *amount* of sleep. Sleep *routine* is equally as important. This means the timing of sleep has to be consistent: getting to sleep and waking up at approximately the same time every day, even on weekends and holidays. If you have difficulty falling asleep, SHARP advocates creating a consistent routine that starts with Pranayama (Complete Breath) before going to bed. You may be surprised at how effective the consistent use of this simple technique can be in improving the quality of your sleep.

This basic technique for proper breathing will help relax your mind and body before bedtime.

1. Find a comfortable position.
2. Sit erect.

3.   Close your eyes.

4.   Inhale steadily through the nostrils for a long deep breath. Do not force your breathing. As you breathe in, focus your attention on the air entering your nose. Feel the cool, calm breath bringing in new, fresh energy and oxygen to your body.

5.   Retain the breath for several seconds.

6.   Exhale very slowly, holding the chest in a firm position. As you exhale, focus your attention on the air as it comes out of your nostrils. Imagine the toxins leaving your body and disappearing into the air, leaving you refreshed and relaxed. Do not force your breath; keep it comfortable.

7.   After completely exhaling, relax the chest and abdomen.

8.   Repeat steps 4 through 7.

Meditation is very effective in quieting the mind and inducing sleep. If your mind is racing or you are worrying a lot, then you need an energetic reset of your autonomic nervous system. Energy healing is very helpful for achieving this.

Relax: Take some time to relax before you go to bed. Have a warm scented bath, read a non-stimulating novel, or have someone give you a gentle massage of the back of your neck and head while you are lying on the bed with your head down. Overall, massage therapy is an excellent way to relax the muscles and relax your mind. It is more than an indulgence. It can be a vital therapy for relaxation and sleep issues.

Stretch it out: If you cannot turn your thoughts off before going to bed, try moderate exercise and stretching before bedtime. This is a great way to wind down the day and prepare for sleep.

Comfort Zone: Make your bedroom a pleasant place to be. Clear it of newspapers, laptops and tablets, and other distractions such as TV. Avoid tobacco, alcohol, or caffeine for at least three to five hours before bedtime.

Stress

Stress management involves more than just relaxation. At its very core, stress management means life management. If all you do is learn relaxation strategies, that is still a Band-Aid approach no matter how helpful those might be. You need to adopt a lifestyle that gives you purpose, satisfaction, and fulfillment. This optimal lifestyle includes rational thinking, positive self-talk, dealing with everyday issues with calm, poise, and acceptance, finding your purpose in life, goal setting, time management, resource management, and problem solving. You need to learn the specialized life skills that will bring success to your life. Total health is not just physical health; it includes mental health, emotional health, spiritual health, financial health, and social health.

Mental and Spiritual Health:

As we saw in the chapter on Laws of Nature, all disease originates in the mind. It is important to determine how you can affect your mind in a positive manner so that it can become health promoting and not disease promoting. How do you accomplish that? How do you change your mind to become health promoting? As we saw in an earlier chapter, the mind is nothing but a repository of your thoughts, and your reality is determined by those thoughts. The easiest way to change your reality is to change your thoughts. However, as you are well aware, that is no easy feat. If it were that simple, there would not be so much suffering in the world.

When a person is physically out of shape, he or she must follow a process to achieve physical fitness. This is also true when one is mentally out of shape. Physical fitness is easy to gauge, as there are objective, measurable parameters that can determine your fitness level. Mental fitness is harder to assess, as the parameters are not as objective. A point of clarification is necessary here. When we talk about mental *fitness*, it should be differentiated from mental *health*, as the term *mental health* is generally used in reference to psychological conditions, such as depression, schizophrenia, and psychosis. What we are discussing here is mental fitness, which refers to the optimal functioning of the mind.

Monitoring Your Headache

All that we have discussed is critical to your success in achieving headache freedom. However, none of that will be possible unless you have a way of tracking and monitoring your progress. The primary goal of this book is to help you control your headaches and your life, and to liberate you from the shackles of dependency on outside measures.

Most headache specialists, clinics, and books ask you to keep a headache journal or diary in which you record your headaches, medications used, and effective lifestyle changes in order to track your progress. While there is no doubt that these headache diaries serve a useful purpose, we suggest you utilize a different approach. As we discussed earlier, an important principle of life is that **what you focus on expands**. If you focus on your headaches, the headaches expand. We want you to focus on optimal health, not on disease or a representation of disease. Just the name *headache journal* signifies to the mind, especially the subconscious mind, that headaches are an important issue for you. The subconscious is very literal in its interpretation of your environment and the data that you put into it. The more you focus on your headaches, the more the subconscious interprets this as something you want, so it gives you more headaches.

Every headache treatment program is unique, because each program is individualized to the needs, circumstances, and goals of each patient. However, there are general principles that serve as guidelines for everyone.

Acute Headaches

All acute headaches need to be treated using whatever approach works best for you. Several options are available including OTC and prescription medications. People adopting SHARP regularly choose acupuncture, massage therapy, mind/body exercises, relaxation, and other stress management exercises instead of medications. They find that quite often they do not need to reach for the ever-present medications, but instead only use them when other choices are not available or feasible.

We suggest the following initial approach to acute headaches:

- Determine what may have caused the acute pain. Have you been under stress lately? If the answer is yes, consider one or more of the following:
  1. Massage therapy
  2. Relaxation

3. Mind-body exercises
4. Physical exercises

- If these measures are not sufficient, the next step is to consider homeopathic medicines and/or herbal treatments for acute pain relief. Acupuncture is a very effective treatment for acute headache.
- If none of the above is effective in controlling the acute pain, medications can be considered. These include OTC non-specific pain medications and prescription medications.
- For relief of acute pain within the setting of chronic pain, the strategy is slightly different. If you are already suffering from chronic headaches, such as migraine headaches, you have most likely been prescribed migraine-specific medications or narcotics. In this situation, we recommend that you should not stop the medications abruptly, but should gradually reduce the dosage under the supervision of a headache specialist, preferably one with experience in alternative strategies. Whatever strategy has worked in the past should be continued, and an individualized plan of chronic pain control should be instituted as detailed below.

These guidelines apply even if you are not taking daily medications for chronic pain. In our experience, a combination of medications and alternative strategies can be very effective in controlling acute pain.

Headache Prevention

When acute headaches become recurrent and more frequent, the condition has become chronic. The strategy for pain control in chronic headaches is different from that of acute pain. SHARP aims to provide you with the various tools that will help you address the cause of the headache while at the same time achieve optimal health. Again, we use whatever approach provides the best prevention, whether it is a medication, an alternative therapy, lifestyle modification, or a combination of the three. Toward this end, the various alternative modalities, such as acupuncture, NAET, massage therapy, nutritional assessment and therapy, homeopathy, and stress management are important aspects of the headache prevention program.

Certain preventative medications can be quite beneficial in obtaining headache relief; however, these medications can cause side effects, so it is important to use them appropriately. We suggest that you consult a headache specialist who is knowledgeable about the appropriate use of these medications. Too often, people comment that they have tried "everything," but further questioning reveals that the medications were not prescribed for an appropriate length of time or the dosage was not appropriate.

Since every individual is unique, it is difficult to provide you with an individualized prescription for chronic headache prevention. However, in order to achieve a true pain-free state, you will have to work with your mind. Until you learn how to shift your focus away from the pain and toward health, the relief will be temporary. The SHARP approach is designed to help you find the most optimal preventative plan for you.

The mainstay of optimal headache prevention is in changing your lifestyle toward a healthier one than you might currently be engaged in. The following is the desired lifestyle that can help you achieve this elusive optimal health by harnessing the powers of nature.

Daily Lifestyle for Optimal Headache Relief

Waking up

Engaging in a few simple routines can set the stage for your day. Quite frequently, many people begin the day after being jolted from sleep by the shrill voice of the alarm clock. This starts the stress hormones pumping even before the first waking moment of the day. Even if you do wake up without the aid of an alarm clock, it would serve you better to take some minutes to sit in a comfortable position and take a few deep breaths to invigorate your body and mind. You may want to meditate for a few minutes. Taking just a few minutes every morning to prepare yourself mentally and relaxing your body and mind helps to start your day with invigorating neurotransmitters propelling you forward rather than stress hormones dragging you down. The morning is the best time to get some cardiovascular exercise, as well as doing meditation and other mind/body exercises. Avoid the typical morning routine of waking up to the alarm clock, listening to the negative news of the world's catastrophes, and sprinting out the door with a cup of coffee in hand. So begins the rat race.

As discussed in the chapter on stress management, the Energizing Alternate Nostril Breathing technique is particularly helpful to bring you fully and peacefully awake. This technique is being provided again for your convenience.

Energizing Alternate Nostril Breathing:
1. Close the right nostril with the thumb of the right hand.
2. Inhale deeply through the left nostril.
3. At the end of the inhalation, let go of the right nostril.
4. Exhale completely through both nostrils.
5. Close the left nostril with the middle finger of the right hand.
6. Then inhale through the right nostril, taking a long deep breath.
7. At the end of the inhalation, let go of the left nostril.
8. Exhale completely through both nostrils.

Breakfast
Breakfast is an important meal of the day, so do not skip it. Keep it relatively simple, consisting of nutritious food that should be easily digestible. Your aim should be to consume food rich in nutrients and balanced in the different food components. Carbohydrates should consist of both simple and complex carbohydrates providing immediate energy as well as slower burning fuel. Add some protein and a small amount of fat. Eating food of differing glycemic indexes will provide a stable source of nutrition all morning long. Avoid the high-fat breakfast typical of the standard American diet consisting of bacon and eggs and a cup of coffee.

We cannot list all the different breakfast options, as everyone's body and diet preferences are unique; however, the following is one example of a healthy breakfast:

1. In-season fresh fruit of your choice
2. A glass of fresh-squeezed orange juice
3. A bowl of steel-cut oatmeal with a touch of honey or maple syrup

My current favorite breakfast is a smoothie made with an apple, orange, pear, strawberries, blueberries, spinach, broccoli, a scoop of flaxseed powder and/ or protein powder. You may question my sanity for drinking a smoothie made with spinach and broccoli for breakfast. However, the presence of so many fruits dilutes the taste of the spinach and broccoli, which means that I am able to eat a handful of fresh, raw, organic spinach leaves with a few florets of raw broccoli without sacrificing the sweet taste of fruit that is so pleasant in the morning. You can substitute frozen fruits and vegetables for fresh ones, especially blueberries, strawberries, broccoli, and others. You can experiment with different types of fruits and vegetables to make your own.

Vitamins and Supplements

Take your vitamins and supplements at the beginning of the day. In today's fast-paced environment, it is almost impossible to get all the essential vitamins and nutrients from diet alone. Most of you will need a multivitamin supplement, but some of you may need more of certain specific nutrients in varying dosages, depending on your particular circumstances. Most of you should be taking extra vitamin B complex, vitamin C, vitamin E, and omega-3 fatty acids, although the majority of you should be taking other vitamins too.

Lunch and Dinner

Make lunch the largest meal of the day. We have found that to be particularly beneficial. Make your dinner smaller than lunch. This will help you to sleep better and control your weight. Reserve your major protein intake for lunch, and make your dinner more carbohydrate-rich.

Stress Reduction

Of paramount importance is managing your stress. This is an integral part of SHARP and should be an important aspect of your headache reduction program as well. There are two ways to manage stress: decrease stress-causing factors and increase relaxation strategies. First, identify the events, circumstances, or people in your life that increase stress; then, devise strategies to minimize your exposure to them. Once you have determined the cause(s) of your stress, the next step is to design ways to minimize the cause(s). The adoption of the five *vital skills* discussed in chapter 21 will be helpful. Treatment strategies need to be tailored to your specific circumstances and coping styles.

You can control stress with quick bouts of relaxation exercises, meditation, and other breathing strategies. You do not have to attend a class on relaxation or yoga to experience their benefit. A few minutes of deep breathing or meditation can elicit the relaxation response quite effectively.

The headache reduction program is about sensible living. It requires a paradigm shift in the way you approach life. Consume foods and engage in activities that will keep you healthy. Stay away from foods and activities that age you faster than your chronological age.

The intensity of the headache determines how aggressive your treatment strategy needs to be. If you suffer from relatively infrequent headaches, then you need the least aggressive treatment. The following chart gives you a general treatment protocol for headache. Of course, this general approach needs to be personalized and individualized depending on your particular circumstances.

Headache Treatment Chart

Treatment Protocol	TTH	Infrequent Migraine	Frequent Migraine		Intractable Headache
Imaging Study (MRI or CT)	If new-onset or very frequent	If new-onset	If new-onset or very frequent		Yes
Dietary Modification	++++	++++	++++		++++
Acute Rx	+	++	++++		++++
Preventative Rx w/ medication	Not necessarily	No	Consider		Most likely
Preventative treatment w/ herbs	Consider +	Consider +++	Consider +++		Consider ++
Control of stressors in lifestyle	++++	++++	++++		++++
Elicitation of relaxation response	++++	++++	++++		++++
Yoga	Yes	Yes	Yes		Yes
Cardiovascular exercise	Yes	Yes	Yes		Yes
Acupuncture	++	++++	++++		++++
NAET	If you have allergies and/or food sensitivities, consider NAET. It is very helpful in decreasing/eliminating headache triggers.				
Homeopathy	++++	++++	++++	++++	
Success Journal	Yes	Yes	Yes		Yes

The next table contains a list of helpful vitamins and nutrients for all headache patients. Other specific nutrients may be beneficial in certain patients, depending on their circumstances.

Helpful Nutrients and Supplements

Nutrient	Recommended dosage	Comments
Multivitamin with minerals	1 tab daily	
Vitamin E	400 units daily	Improves circulation Use the d-alpha-tocopherol form
Calcium	1500 mg daily	Helps to alleviate muscular tension
Magnesium	100 mg daily	Deficiency may cause migraines
Coenzyme Q10	100 mg daily or more	
Glucosamine	1500 mg daily	An alternative to NSAIDs
B complex vitamins	At least 50 mg of each major B vitamin twice daily, except as noted below	Helps in the optimal functioning of the brain and nerves, especially if under stress
Extra B-2 (Riboflavin)	400 mg daily	Helpful in migraine prevention
Folic acid	800 microgram daily	
Vitamin B-12	500 microgram daily	
Vitamin C with bioflavonoids	2000 to 8000 mg daily in divided doses	Helps protect against harmful effects of pollution and stress
Essential fatty acid complex	As directed on label	

This list is by no means comprehensive, as there are many more nutrients being discovered on a regular basis. It can serve as a basic guide to the key ingredients that should be part of any headache reduction program.

People report benefits within days to weeks. Of course, if you are suffering only from infrequent headaches, and you treat your headache with appropriate medication, you will experience significant improvement in a matter of minutes to a few hours. When we talk about benefits, we are interested in improving your overall health and preventing your headaches. The first noticeable improvement might be in your energy level. You will most likely notice increased physical energy, which is generally due to the improved efficiency of your brain chemicals and neurotransmitters, and normalization of your vitamin levels.

This is usually followed by an improvement in your emotional well-being. The disability from chronic headache will also start to improve, which is characterized by decrease in the frequency, intensity, and duration of the chronic pain. Soon you will experience an improvement in your higher cognitive functions, such as memory and concentration. Your daily productivity will improve, accompanied by a higher level of satisfaction and fulfillment, ultimately leading to a happier, higher quality of life.

Headache Freedom Plan

In order to achieve headache freedom, you have to design a program that is unique to you, as your circumstances are unique to you. If you have been taking notes and doing the action exercises at the end of each chapter, you have already started designing your treatment plan for headache freedom.

The answers to the following questions will help you to design your own **Nine Steps to Headache Freedom:**

1. What do I want my life to be like?
2. What are the most important things in my life?
3. What are my triggers?
4. Am I a stressful person? What causes me stress? What was my Stress Impact Index? What is my Stress Type?
5. Do I sleep well? Do I wake up refreshed?
6. Am I willing to take medications to stop the pain?
7. Do I have any health conditions that may affect the choice of medications?
8. Am I truly healthy according to the positive indicators of health mentioned in Chapter 17?
9. Am I willing to try acupuncture and homeopathy?

246 | Not Tonight I Have a HEADACHE

10. Do I have sensitivities/allergies?

11. Am I willing to spend time on relaxation strategies?

12. Am I willing to change my lifestyle to achieve headache freedom?

Nine Steps to Headache Freedom

The action exercises and the answers to the preceding questions will help you to design your own personalized **Nine Steps to Headache Freedom:**

1. Acute therapy:

_____

2. Preventative therapy:

_____

3. Acupuncture/Homeopathy:

_____

4. Exercise Plan:

_____

5. Relaxation Plan:

_____

6. Nutrition plan with allergy elimination:

_____

7. Supplements:

_____

8. Yoga:

_____

9. My Life Purpose:

_____

APPENDICES

Life-Threatening Causes of Secondary Headaches

Medical conditions causing secondary headaches	
Head trauma	Brain hemorrhage: epidural, subdural, subarachnoid After brain surgery (post-craniotomy)
Vascular disorder	Stroke, TIA Non-traumatic brain hemorrhage of all types Arterio-venous malformation (AVM) Dural arterio-venous fistula Giant cell arteritis Vertebral artery pain (due to dissection)
Non-vascular intracranial disorder	Idiopathic intracranial hypertension Hydrocephalus Low intracranial pressure Brain tumor (neoplasm) Non-infectious inflammatory diseases (neurosarcoid, aseptic meningitis) Post-seizure headache
Substance use or its withdrawal	Nitrous oxide (NO) Carbon monoxide (CO) Alcohol-induced Monosodium glutamate (MSG) Cocaine Medication over-use
Infection	Bacterial meningitis Viral meningitis Brain abscess HIV/AIDS

Disorder of homeostasis	Post-dialysis
	Driving headache
	Hypertension-induced
	Hypertensive encephalopathy
	Eclampsia
	Fasting

APPENDIX 2

Common OTC Medications

Brand Name	Generic Name	Dosage	Common Uses	Common Side Effects
Anacin Bayer Bufferin Ecotrin Midol	Aspirin	325 mg	Minor aches, pains, and headache	Aspirin allergy, asthma, upset stomach, Reye's Syndrome
Anacin-3 Excedrin Tylenol	Acetaminophen	500 mg	Headache	May cause liver damage
Advil Motrin Nuprin Medipren	Ibuprofen	200 mg	Fever and muscle ache	Aspirin allergy, asthma, upset stomach, not for last trimester
Aleve Naprosyn	Naproxen Sodium	220 mg	Musculoskeletal	Higher heart attack risk, upset stomach, not for nursing mothers
Motrin 800	Ibuprofen	800 mg	Fever and muscle ache	Aspirin allergy, asthma, upset stomach, not for last trimester
Excedrin Extra-strength	Acetaminophen aspirin caffeine	250 mg250 mg 65 mg	Minor aches, pains, and headache	Aspirin allergy, asthma, upset stomach, Reye's Syndrome
Excedrin Tension	Acetaminophen caffeine	500 mg, 65 mg	Ttension headaches	May cause liver damage
Excedrin Migraine	Acetaminophen aspirin caffeine	250 mg, 250 mg, 65 mg	Migraine headaches	Aspirin allergy, asthma, upset stomach, Reye's Syndrome

| Extra-strength Tylenol | Acetaminophen | 500 mg | Headache and other minor aches | May cause liver damage |

Non-Specific Prescription Headache Medications

Brand Name	Generic Name	Dosage	Features and Common Uses	Common Side Effects
Motrin 800	Ibuprofen	800 mg	fever, muscle ache	Aspirin allergy, asthma, upset stomach, not for last trimester
Voltaren, Voltaren-XR	Diclofenac	25 mg, 50 mg, 75 mg, 100 mg	a stronger NSAID	Gastro-intestinal ulcerations, abdominal burning, pain, cramping, nausea, gastritis, and even serious gastrointestinal bleeding and liver toxicity
Kadian	Morphine	20 mg, 30 mg, 50 mg, 60 mg, 100 mg	Migraine headaches	Constipation, lightheadedness, dizziness, drowsiness, stomach upset, nausea, and flushing the first few days
Oxycontin	Oxycodone	5 mg, 10 mg, 20 mg, 40 mg	Narcotic pain reliever and cough suppressant	Lightheadedness, dizziness, sedation, nausea, and vomiting
Darvon	Propoxyphene	65 mg	Two-thirds as potent as codeine	Lightheadedness, dizziness, sedation, nausea, and vomiting

Vicodin, Vicodin ES Percocet Lortab Lorcet Norco	Hydrocodone and Acetaminophen	2.5 mg to 10 mg 500 mg to 750 mg	Weakest of the narcotics	Lightheadedness, dizziness, sedation, nausea, vomiting, and difficulty urinating
Ultram	Tramadol	50 mg	Non-narcotic, but stronger than Hydrocodone, less potential for abuse and addiction	Nausea, constipation, dizziness, headache, drowsiness, and vomiting
Demerol	Meperidine		Moderate to severe pain	Stomach upset, blurred vision, drowsiness, constipation, dizziness or lightheadedness

Common Triptans in Use for Acute Treatment

Brand name (Generic) and Formulations	Features and Side Effects
Imitrex (Sumatriptan) Tablet (25 mg, 50 mg, 100 mg) Injection (4 mg, 6 mg) Nasal spray (5 mg, 10 mg)	First triptan introduced; also used for cluster headaches Nausea, dizziness, tingling of the skin, drowsiness, neck or throat tightness, jaw pain
Zomig (Zolmitriptan) Tablet (2.5 mg, 5 mg) ZMT (oral melttabs)	Has faster onset and may be more effective Nausea, dizziness, tingling of the skin, drowsiness, neck or throat tightness, jaw pain
Amerge (Naratriptan) Tablet (1 mg and 2.5 mg)	Fewer side effects (mainly nausea and vomiting), and lasts longer to reduce recurrence; best choice for migraine recurrence and menstrual migraine
Maxalt (Rizatriptan) Tablet (5 mg and 10 mg) Orally dissolving (5 mg and 10 mg)	Also helps nausea, vomiting, light and sound sensitivity Bitter taste, dizziness, sleepiness, nausea
Treximet (Sumatriptan and Naproxen) Sumatriptan 85 mg and Naproxen 500 mg	Combination of two medications with different actions; more effective than either agent alone; specific for migraine
Axert (Almotriptan) Tablet (6.25 mg and 12.5 mg)	Contains a sulfa drug, so should not be used in patients allergic to sulfonamides

Frova (Frovatriptan) Tablet (2.5 mg)	Long-acting triptan; also works well for menstrual migraine Can cause dizziness, fatigue, dry mouth
Relpax (Eletriptan) Tablet (20 mg and 40 mg)	More effective in the short-term Weakness, upset stomach, heartburn

Results of the Twenty-Year Study on Stress Management Conducted by the Canadian Institute of Stress

Program Results at Four and Eight Months Follow-Up		
	At 4 months	At 8 months
Doctor's office visits decrease	22%	53%
Days absent from work decrease	42%	58%
Below target blood pressure	49%	91%
Immunoglobulin A increase	24%	31%
T cell increase	16%	28%
Stress hyper-reactivity down	41%	46%
Stress recovery time down	28%	36%
Ability to relax at will increase	17%	31%

What they also found was that it is important to identify which types of patients need help the most and are likely to experience the greatest benefit from stress management techniques. They divided people according to where they were on a continuum:

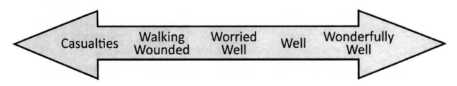

Casualties Walking Wounded Worried Well Well Wonderfully Well

As a general rule, patients who fall into the category of *well* and *wonderfully well* may not need any specific stress management techniques, as their stress level, as defined above, does not produce negative consequences.

The patients we are more concerned with are the ones who fall into the other three categories:

The *walking wounded* are those patients who have chronically elevated stress, as indicated by physical problems such as fatigue, headache, muscle tension/spasm, sleep disturbance, generalized anxiety, difficulties or reduced satisfaction in relationships, depressed mood, motivation or enthusiasm, frequent and/or unusually prolonged minor illnesses, as well as stress exacerbating other conditions (arthritis, allergies, skin problems).

The *worried well* are those for whom frequent recurring periods of high stress are interfering with health, or with their satisfaction and participation in relationships, work/career, or personal life.

The *casualties* are those patients who need more appropriate medical or other professional referral, for whom revitalization is a major aim in the treatment of a diagnosed illness or problem in living (sleep disorder, addiction, anxiety or panic attack, disruptive career change).

APPENDIX 6

Diet Modification and Migraine Recurrence

In the study on the lifestyle modification approach to headache treatment, Dr. Bic examined the role of changing a person's lifestyle on headache recurrence. The study was conducted over a period of twelve weeks; however, the first four weeks were spent collecting the baseline information, and intervention was started at the end of the four weeks.

Table: Results of the Migraine Headache Prevention Study

Migraine headache characteristics studied	At baseline (prior to intervention)	At study end	Result
Headache frequency (in a 4-week period)	9 episodes	2 episodes	Improvement of nearly 71%
Headache intensity (on a scale of 1-5, with 5 being the worst headache)	3	<1	Decrease of 66%
Migraine headache duration	As measured by a special measure called the Headache Index		Decrease of 74%
Medication intake	Approximately 10 times per month	3 times per month	Decrease of 72%
Overall results	94% of patients reported at least a 40% improvement		

Types of Fats

Saturated fats	Monounsaturated fats	Polyunsaturated fats
Beef	Avocado	Almonds
Butter	Canola oil	Corn oil/Cottonseed oil
Cheese	Cashews	Fish
Chocolate/Cocoa butter	Olives/olive oil	Mayonnaise
Coconut/Coconut oil	Peanuts/Peanut butter	Pecans
Cream	Peanut oil	Safflower/Soybean oil
Lamb		Sesame seeds/Sesame oil
Lard		Sunflower seeds
Milk		Sunflower oil
Pork		Walnuts
Poultry		
Palm oil		

About the Author

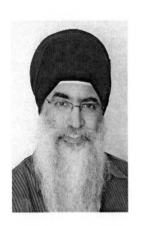

Ravinder Singh, MD, SWC
Diplomate, American Board of Psychiatry and Neurology
Certified Stress and Wellness Consultant
Beverly Hills Headache Institute
8920 Wilshire Blvd., Suite 520
Beverly Hills, CA 90212
Telephone: (310) 432-2880, Fax: (310) 432-2887
Email: drsingh@bhhi1.com
www.bhhi1.com

Dr. Ravinder Singh is a board-certified neurologist specializing in the prevention and treatment of neurological diseases, especially stroke, headache, and epilepsy.

Ravinder Singh received his medical degree in 1989 from St. George's University, School of Medicine, in Grenada, West Indies. He completed his Neurology residency at West LA VA Medical Center/UCLA in Los Angeles, California. In 1994, he became Chief Resident in Neurology, subsequently followed by a VA Fellowship grant in Neuroscience and Traumatic Brain

Injuries. During this time, he also became a Clinical Instructor in Neurology at University of California, Los Angeles (UCLA). After completing his training, he became an Assistant Professor of Neuroscience at Charles R. Drew University of Medicine and Science, and Head of the Stroke Center at King-Drew Medical Center, in Los Angeles, California. He has served as the President of the American Heart Association, LA division. He is currently in private practice in Beverly Hills, California.

Dr. Singh established **Beverly Hills Headache Institute**, a unique integrative facility that employs a team of highly qualified experts from the ancient Eastern healing traditions such as Ayurveda and Traditional Chinese Medicine to the distinguished physicians practicing modern medical sciences. Integrating the best of Western and Eastern approaches in the prevention of disease, Beverly Hills Headache Institute creates customized treatment plans for the optimal health of its clients.

Dr. Singh is also a Certified Stress and Wellness Consultant. He utilizes his knowledge of Western and Eastern medicine, as well as his studies in stress and wellness medicine to help people achieve greater satisfaction in their lives and achieve long-lasting optimal health, with an emphasis on disease prevention. He provides individualized yet systematic solutions that are leading edge, scientifically based, and proven in the real world. These very pragmatic and results-oriented solutions and skills are immediately applicable and geared toward high-speed success.

Dr. Singh has given over 100 presentations on the topics of stress management, stroke, headache, and epilepsy to the medical community. He has been an invited lecturer and presenter at over 100 hospitals and other related organizations in the United States. He has been the **featured speaker** on the topic of Stroke at the regional board meetings for the American Heart Association. He has also been the spokesperson for the **Train to End Stroke** program of the American Stroke Association. In addition, Dr. Singh has made many media appearances, including mainstream and cable television and radio networks.

He is married and lives in Culver City, California.

CPSIA information can be obtained at www.ICGtesting.com
Printed in the USA
LVOW10s1729200715

446921LV00006B/534/P